Who's hungry? And how do we know?

Who's hungry? And how do we know? Food shortage, poverty, and deprivation

Laurie DeRose, Ellen Messer, and Sara Millman

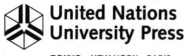

United Nations University Press

TOKYO · NEW YORK · PARIS

United Nations University Press
The United Nations University, 53-70, Jingumae 5-chome, Shibuya-ku, Tokyo 150, Japan
Tel: (03) 3499-2811   Fax: (03) 3406-7345
E-mail: mbox@hq.unu.edu

UNU Office in North America
2 United Nations Plaza, Room DC2-1462-70, New York, NY 10017
Tel: (212) 963-6387   Fax: (212) 371-9454   Telex: 422311 UN UI

United Nations University Press is the publishing division of the United Nations University.

Cover design by J.-M. Antenen, Geneva

Printed in the United States of America

UNUP-985
ISBN 92-808-0985-7

    DeRose, Laurie Fields, 1968–
    Who's hungry? And how do we know? : food shortage, poverty, and deprivation / Laurie DeRose, Ellen Messer, and Sara Millman.
        p. cm.
    Includes bibliographical references and index.
    ISBN 9280809857 (pbk.)
    1. Poverty. 2. Hunger. 3. Starvation. 4. Food supply.
    5. Nutrition policy. 6. Famines. 7. War and society.
    8. Economic sanctions. I. Messer, Ellen.
    II. Millman, Sara. III. Title.
      HC79.P6D47   1998
      363.8—dc21
    97-45294
    CIP

Contents

Contents

Preface

In July 1986 the Feinstein World Hunger Program faculty at Brown University, directed by geographer Robert Kates, began formulating a conceptual framework for analysing hunger and hunger-related policy making. This "hunger typology" is based on a three-tiered paradigm of hunger causation and consequences that draws on methods of food production/famine research, entitlement theory, and nutrition/nutritional anthropology. The framework brings together the disparate disciplines of political economics, sociology–anthropology, and public health–human biology, and also policy and organizational research. It integrates their approaches and evidence into a single format that allows all to identify "who's hungry" and take steps to prevent and alleviate hunger.

The hunger typology distinguishes among situations of *food shortage*, *food poverty*, or *food deprivation*. At a regional or national level, a food shortage may be due to political, climatic, or other socioeconomic forces. Such food-short or famine conditions can be distinguished from food poverty at the household level, in which people go hungry because they lack the resources to acquire food even when the regional food supply is sufficient. Ultimately, even if households have sufficient resources to command and access food, individuals go hungry if distribution rules militate against their getting an adequate share, if cultural rules of consumption prejudice them from consuming an adequate mix of nutrients, or if individuals are ill and unable to ingest, metabolize, or benefit from the nutrients potentially available. This third context, termed food deprivation, includes situations of malnutrition among the so-called vulnerable groups: infants and young children, pregnant and lactating women, and others who are deprived of food in situations of social powerlessness or illness.

Sara Millman, a sociologist–demographer associated with the World Hunger Program, proposed in 1988 that the United Nations University sponsor a project that would review the evidence for hunger of each category, and offered to prepare a manual reviewing the data. Her student and colleague, Laurie DeRose, also a demographer–sociologist, in 1995 assumed the lead in completing the project. She drew on Millman's initial outline and also her drafts for chapters 1 (the framework), 2 (methods of measurement), and 5 (food deprivation); drafted chapter 4 (food poverty), and wrote chapter 3 (food shortage) with additional assistance from myself. I also wrote the separate chapter on conflict, which highlights its significance as a source of hunger.

The chapters together illustrate the utility of the hunger typology for diagnosing hunger vulnerability of countries, regions, households, and individuals, and also discusses the reliability of the methods used to measure or indicate each type of hunger and its principal causes. Using this framework, it is possible to profile the incidence of different types of hunger in any single location or year, as the World Hunger Program has done in its biannual *Hunger Report* series. It is also possible to arrive at local or global histories of hunger, as the World Hunger Program did in *Hunger in History* (Basil Blackwell, 1990), edited by Lucile Newman.

We are very happy to be able to add this volume to our series of publications that use the hunger typology as a framework for scholarly research, policy diagnosis, and practical action to prevent and alleviate hunger.

Ellen Messer
Director
Alan Shawn Feinstein World Hunger Program

Acknowledgements

Several people have been instrumental in allowing this project to be completed. We would like to thank especially Abraham Besrat, Director of the Development Studies Program at the United Nations University (Tokyo), for his encouragement and patience throughout the duration of this project. We would also like to thank Robert Kates, who was the initial instigator and early on provided advice and encouragement, and Monica Das Gupta, who worked and generously shared her data with Sara Millman.

1

Introduction

Laurie F. DeRose and Sara R. Millman

Framework: Food shortage, food poverty, food deprivation

Any attempt to reduce hunger requires a sound understanding of which people are affected. The answer to the question "who's hungry?" matters because hunger is both damaging and avoidable. This volume answers the question at three basic levels of social organization: it identifies hungry regions, hungry households within regions, and hungry individuals within households. Vulnerability to hunger is not distributed evenly at any of these levels, and whether vulnerability results in hunger also depends on the way people organize themselves in relation to hunger.

Differentiating between production shortfalls on a regional level (food shortage), inadequate food availability within a household (food poverty), and individual malnutrition (food deprivation) makes it easier to identify the hungry; more importantly, it helps highlight the type of problem leading to hunger. Production difficulties and distribution inequities require different types of solutions, and effectively combating hunger requires finding solutions that address the actual problems. Knowing who is hungry moves us closer to workable solutions.

The framework used in this book (see fig. 1.1) distinguishing food shortage, food poverty, and food deprivation does not assume that "the real problem" lies at one of these three levels. We have not adopted a strong theoretical view that dictates that efforts to reduce hunger need to be focused primarily on one type of intervention. Instead, our framework is designed to call attention to hunger even when food is abundant, as well as to learn how hunger is avoided even when food is scarce.

Part of our task is to show the complex relationships between hunger at the different levels of social organization. The remainder of this chapter outlines the links between these types of hunger and it also overviews the manifestations of hunger in order to show that hunger has consequences, as well as causes, specific to each of the levels of social organization.

Links between levels of hunger

Hunger is produced when need outstrips food availability, but the determinants of both need and availability are complex: they are controlled by forces both proximate to and quite remote from the individuals they affect. In food shortage, food supplies within some bounded region are less than the amount needed by the region's population. In food poverty, a household is unable to obtain enough food to meet the needs of its members. And in food deprivation, the nutrients consumed by an individual are less than he or she needs.

The three situations are causally linked, as shown in figure 1.1. One reason for food deprivation is food poverty, and one reason for food poverty is food shortage. It may seem obvious that if there is not enough food in the region some households will not have enough, and if there is not enough food in the household some members will go hungry. But it is also true that in food-short areas some households are more than adequately provisioned, and in non-food-short areas, some households are not able to meet the needs of all of their members. There are many possible causes of food poverty and deprivation other than food shortage.

The distinction among the three levels of social organization is helpful in considering which of the many different causes of hunger may be at work in any particular case and in avoiding the fallacious view of hunger as a single, simple problem. It also provides a framework within which the insights of disciplines focusing on one or another of the levels, and the distinctive policy foci of various organizations, may be integrated.

This can easily be seen by considering famine conditions – those in which widespread severe food shortage had led to elevated mortality and mass movements of populations in search of food. Famine has often been viewed as a production failure. Many international food aid efforts focus on simply increasing the supply of food available in

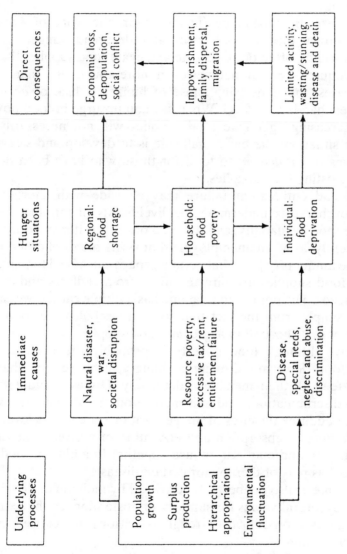

Fig. 1.1 A causal structure of hunger (source: Newman et al. 1990)

3

such situations. A similar concern for the adequacy of aggregate food supplies in the longer term motivated the work of Green Revolution scientists to increase productive capacity in agriculture after World War II and is among the concerns driving current research in agro-biotechnology.

Recent research on famine (in particular, the work of Amartya Sen) has shown that massive crises of widespread hunger and increased mortality often occur despite aggregate food supplies that are no less adequate – and sometimes even more abundant – than usual. In such cases, the underlying cause of hunger is lack of *access* to food rather than lack of food. When such an upsurge in food poverty occurs, increasing aggregate food supplies will not necessarily improve the situation; the basic challenge is to develop and safeguard mechanisms of *entitlement* to food for those who have been denied access to existing food supplies.

Widespread entitlement failure may coincide with shortage, as when poor harvests undermine the livelihoods of farmers, reduce aggregate food availability, and drive up prices. Or it may occur quite independently, as when unemployment or rising prices of other goods reduce the amounts of food that certain groups can afford to purchase, or when food supplies are directed away from civilians and toward military needs. The point is that famine has multiple causes: we cannot conclude simply from the fact that some households are food poor that there is any shortfall in aggregate food supply.

Similarly, although food poverty is probably the most obvious cause of food deprivation, many go hungry in households that can afford to feed all their members adequately. Disease, voluntary abstention, discrimination, and misunderstood nutritional needs are among the additional causes of hunger that operate at this level.

Disease impairs absorption and utilization of nutrients, raises nutritional needs, and may also reduce appetite. In addition, food may be withheld as part of therapy for certain diseases.

Food intake is also deliberately restricted by individuals desiring to conform to cultural values for slimness or abstention. In the extreme, hunger strikes for political or religious reasons are carried to the point of starvation.

In households that can afford to feed all their members, discriminatory patterns of food allocation may give some more than they need and others less; where household food supplies are scant, such patterns may leave favoured members adequately fed and deprive others disproportionately. Although it is tempting to interpret this pattern as reflecting a deliberate decision to favour one and deprive the other, variations in the adequacy of the diet of members of the same household may also result from a misunderstanding of need. The nutritional difficulties of young children and pregnant women are cases in point. A child may become malnourished despite being given as much as he or she will eat, if the need for a more nutrient-dense diet is not recognized. Although this problem frequently arises in cultures whose diet is based on starchy staples – toddlers do not have the stomach capacity to eat enough of such foods to satisfy their caloric needs – it has parallels in societies with more diverse diets: parents in the United States have to be taught not to give skim milk to children under two. Similarly, nutritional needs during pregnancy may be under-appreciated by women who believe that delivery of a small baby will be less difficult and thus deliberately restrict their intake during pregnancy. Automatic interpretation of all differences in the adequacy of individual diets within households as discrimination, inappropriately classifies problems caused by disease, household survival strategies, or misunderstood need and could easily lead to ineffective interventions.

At each of these three levels, vulnerability to hunger, its social distribution, and corrective response clearly have a political dimension. The explicit or implicit promise of food security comprises an essential aspect of the social contract between political leaders and their constituents. An end to hunger cannot come about without political leaders who make ending hunger a priority and devote resources to this end (Barraclough 1989). Politicians are important social actors shaping the economic, social, and cultural framework for community organization. Specific descriptions of political obligations are also contained in the emergent concept of the human right to food (Messer 1996; Oshaug et al. 1994).

Why hunger matters

The significance of hunger lies primarily in the damage it does to those who suffer it, and secondarily in the ramifications of efforts made to avoid it. Figure 1.1 shows how some of the consequences at the individual level can easily lead to extreme changes at the other levels of social organization. This figure is a great oversimplification of both the causes and consequences of hunger but it helps highlight

5

some of the significant relationships between hunger and human development, including the impact of hunger on the environment, economic growth, health and family planning, and political order.

Some of the possible consequences of food shortage, food poverty, and food deprivation are presented below, along with further explication of the causal relationships between these consequences. We begin with a relatively lengthy discussion of the effects of food deprivation, in order to increase awareness of how devastating hunger is for the individual; this in turn will facilitate understanding of how individual hunger profoundly affects the social order. This is clear from the conceptual framework.

Effects of hunger on the individual

We define individual hunger as consumption of a diet insufficient to support normal growth, health, and activity. This definition leaves open questions of whether norms are fixed across populations and over time, and of what nutritional requirements are associated with them. These questions, each the subject of considerable controversy, are discussed in subsequent chapters. In the sense we use the term, hunger does not necessarily imply appetite. Individuals may eat enough of certain bulky diets to feel satiated and yet obtain fewer calories and less of some or all nutrients than they need, while those who eat enough of a more nutrient-dense diet to satisfy their appetites may also be malnourished and vulnerable to diet-related chronic disease: excessive fat is growing as a dietary problem in urban communities in developing countries. The physiological effects of hunger vary according to the particular nutrient(s) deficient (or in excess) in the diet and also the age, health, and reproductive status of the individual. The discussion below focuses first on protein–energy malnutrition and then turns to micronutrient deficiencies. Variations in the impact of malnutrition over the life cycle are taken up in the following section on effects of hunger on the household.

Protein–energy malnutrition

The combined insufficiency of calories and protein, or protein–energy malnutrition (PEM), is now considered to be the most widespread form of hunger. Although protein deficiency – including its severe clinical form, kwashiorkor – was once considered the predominant form of undernutrition, nutritionists now agree that most traditional vegetarian diets, consumed in quantities sufficient to meet energy needs, generally provide adequate protein as well, even where animal foods are absent.

Nevertheless, some of those subsisting on largely grain- or tuber-based diets may be at risk of protein deficiency. Young children (particularly weanlings) need more nutrient-dense, protein-rich foods because of their smaller intake capacities. There is mounting evidence that, even if weaning foods are eaten in sufficient quantity to meet energy requirements, there may be important protein and micronutrient deficiencies (Allen et al. 1991; Brown 1991; Golden and Golden 1991; McGuire 1991; Pollitt 1991; West 1991).

Protein quality may also be a problem for poorer segments of the population who may not be able to afford the more expensive non-grain elements in traditional combinations of vegetable foods that together make complete proteins. If they must subsist on only grain, rather than roots or grains with a complementary sauce or garnish (or with another vegetable food that provides the rest of the amino acids to make a complete protein), the quality of protein available to them is less satisfactory. The manifestations of severe protein deficiency overlap with conditions caused by inadequate caloric intake, but protein deficiency carries with it additional problems from fat accumulation in the liver, oedema, and severe anaemia (Hamilton et al. 1985).

When diets are also inadequate in energy, individuals adjust by reducing expenditures through curtailment of physical activity. This behavioural shift has an emotional analogue in apathy (including reduced appetite) and irritability. The costs are obviously reductions in work, in socializing, and, for children, in the interaction with their environment that contributes to their learning and development.

Some physiological adaptation to scarcity also occurs: the basal metabolic rate, or use of energy to power such basic and essential life processes as respiration and circulation, is reduced. But such adaptations have limits that vary across individuals and possibly within individuals over time; causes of this variation are not well understood. These should be viewed as "adjustments" to scarcity that are made at some cost to the well-being of most individuals.

Another consequence of low energy intakes is reduced growth (in children) or weight loss. Energy expenditure may be maintained at a level in excess of consumption by metabolizing reserves in the form of stored body fat. Later, lean body mass in the form of muscle and even organ tissue will also be consumed if inadequate intake persists. Weight loss accompanies the initial stages of inadequate energy intake but, if prolonged, is followed by wasting – in its severe clinical form, marasmus. Death from starvation is the ultimate outcome where intake less than expenditure continues long enough. However, most hunger-related deaths are due to infectious disease rather than starvation *per se*: with severe malnutrition, ability to resist infection deteriorates sharply.

The relationship between malnutrition and infection is a reciprocal and synergistic one. Disease leads to a deterioration in nutritional status at the same time that malnutrition increases susceptibility to disease. Effects of disease on nutritional status involve shifts in the types and quantities of foods consumed (whether due to custom or loss of appetite) and to decreased absorption and diarrhoea. Parasitic organisms, as in malaria or schistosomiasis, or intestinal worms, divert nutrients for their own use. Energy, protein, and micronutrient needs are elevated in order to fight off infection. Immune function also deteriorates with extreme PEM; evidence is more mixed as to possible increases in susceptibility to infection with mild to moderate malnutrition.

Functionally, we observe the effect of sustained hunger far short of starvation largely as lethargy. Ability to carry out heavy manual labour is impaired; the periods over which substantial physical effort can be maintained are reduced. An undernourished manual worker is likely to be less productive than a well-nourished one, to need longer breaks between periods of effort, to be able to work fewer hours per day, and to need to spend more of his non-working time resting. Even aside from performance on the job, the restriction of physical activity clearly implies a reduced quality of life.

In children, the additional effects of even mild to moderate PEM are delayed or permanently stunted growth and higher morbidity and, ultimately, mortality. Although public health statistics tend to ascribe child deaths to either malnutrition or infectious disease, such causes tend to be interlinked. Quantifying the interaction for a series of case studies from developing countries, David Pelletier concluded that malnutrition contributed to 56 per cent of all child deaths, owing to its potentiating effect on infectious disease. About 83 per cent of these malnutrition-related deaths were attributed to mild-to-moderate malnutrition (Pelletier 1994). These findings highlight the magnitude of the problem of food deprivation as a contributor to mortality in young children. Elevated morbidity and mortality are also associated with micronutrient malnutrition, especially vitamin A and iron deficiencies.

Micronutrient deficiencies

Even if food is consumed in quantities sufficient to meet both caloric and protein needs, requirements for various vitamins and minerals may go unsatisfied. Three major micronutrient deficiencies are considered important public health problems today, meaning both that they affect large numbers of people and that their consequences are severe: these are deficiencies of iron, iodine, and vitamin A. Specific micronutrient deficiencies are associated with distinct problems in health and function.

Iron deficiency is believed to be the most common micronutrient deficiency in the world today. It appears, from incomplete evidence, to be most common in South Asia and Africa. About 22 per cent of the world's population is thought to have deficiencies of iron extreme enough to cause anaemia (Ralte 1996). Iron deficiency is especially common among reproductive-aged women, whose requirements are higher than those of others. Although traditional diets throughout most of the world seem to provide large amounts of iron, its biological availability varies according to source. Iron from animal sources is relatively well absorbed (that from human milk best of all); that from grains and vegetables less so. Parasites that divert the body's iron to their own use and/or cause faecal blood loss may also produce iron deficiency.

Iron is used in the transport of oxygen in the blood, and most of the problems associated with its deficiency relate to inadequate supplies of oxygen reaching the cells in which it is needed. Even mild deficiencies of iron seem to be associated with lack of physical energy and difficulties in concentration, with resulting losses of work productivity for adults and of education for children. Iron deficiency anaemia, although common, is increasingly recognized as only the most extreme form of a nutritional problem affecting many more people. Anaemia and subclinical iron deficiency are products and markers of impoverished, unhygienic, and unhealthy environments. Long-term consequences of iron deficiency tend to perpetuate poverty by reducing physical and cognitive development and function of those that are iron deprived.

The next most common micronutrient deficiency is iodine deficiency, with an estimated 655 million cases of goitre (Millman et al. 1991; Ralte 1996) and almost 6 million cretins worldwide (Grant 1995). The most severe problem is geographically restricted to areas with iodine-poor soils that are typically mountainous, glaciated, and/or subject to heavy rainfall or flooding. Milder forms may occur in these and other regions (including industrially developed European countries) where intakes of iodine-adequate foods are low. Goitrogenic substances may also induce iodine deficiency despite apparently good iodine supply. Where soil has inadequate amounts of iodine, insufficient amounts are present both in plants and in animals fed on those plants. Within affected areas, deficiency is most common for those whose diet is most restricted to locally grown foods. Consumption of imported foods tends to be protective. Where locally grown foods are cheaper, we also may expect an association of iodine deficiency with poverty within affected regions. The greatest concentrations of population in areas of iodine deficiency are found in South-East Asia, although there are also pockets of severely affected populations in Africa and Latin America.

Effects of this iodine deficiency disease are both physical and mental. Cretinism, which is irreversible, results from severe iodine deficiency during gestation. The condition combines "profound mental deficiency, a characteristic appearance, a shuffling gait, and a spastic dysphagia" (Scrimshaw 1990). Goitre, a pronounced swelling of the thyroid gland, may develop at any time. High rates of milder mental impairment have been found in areas in which goitre and cretinism occur, and it is now believed that those visibly affected are only a fraction of those whose function is impaired. UNICEF has estimated that 30 per cent of the world's population is at risk of mental and physical impairment due to iodine deficiency, even though less than half of that number manifest signs of goitre or cretinism (Grant 1995). According to one authority (Stanbury 1991), "Iodine deficiency is the most frequent cause of preventable mental retardation today."

Deficiency of vitamin A was estimated to affect some 231 million children in 1994 (Grant 1995), over half of them in just three countries – Bangladesh, India, and Indonesia. Vitamin A is provided by a wide range of vegetable and animal sources but children, especially, may lack adequate access, owing to culture or economic restrictions in diet.

Vitamin A deficiency is a major cause of blindness, mainly in childhood. Many of those blinded die shortly thereafter. It has also been linked to greatly increased vulnerability to infectious disease, with some studies claiming dramatic reduction in child mortality when vitamin A supplementation is provided to all children in areas in which even a few show the visible signs of vitamin A deficiency. Controversy continues on the linkage to mortality from infectious disease (Hussey and Klein 1990; Ramachandran 1991; Rathmathullah et al. 1990). However, most authorities seem to agree that, in at least some populations, vitamin A deficiency is a major contributor to high death rates in childhood. Even mild vitamin A deficiency has been associated with increased vulnerability to respiratory infections, diarrhoea, and complications of measles, all of which are major causes of death among children in many less-developed countries (Tomkins and Watson 1989).

Other micronutrient deficiencies are less common than these three but may be significant in certain populations or settings. Pellagra, beriberi, scurvy, and rickets, associated respectively with deficiencies of niacin, thiamine, vitamin C, and vitamin D, were important public health problems in the past but are now relatively rare. They are sometimes observed, however, among refugee populations subsisting on food aid rations based on an unusually restricted range of foods (Chen 1990). In addition, zinc deficiency lately is becoming recognized as a significant contributing factor to poor health and growth, although the absence of a reliable index of human zinc deficiency and of obvious clinical features make diagnosis and assessment of impairments uncertain (Cousins and Hempe 1990).

Detailed data on the prevalence of these micronutrient deficiencies in specific groups and locations are scarce and unstandardized, and they will not be explored further in this volume. Overall, recent advances in the study of each of the major micronutrient deficiencies suggest that effects are far more widely distributed than previously believed and that the subtler and less visible effects of milder forms of iron deficiency, iodine deficiency, and vitamin A deficiency on mental function and vulnerability to disease may dwarf their more easily identified manifestations in total impact. Increasing attention to these problems will add to our store of knowledge about who is affected.

Effects of hunger on the household

Households with hungry members face limitations that affect both their current daily activities and their longer-term welfare. Hungry mothers are less able to nourish and care for their children, maintain household functioning, and provide additional household resources to improve nutrition. Hungry workers generally earn less and have less energy for household maintenance activities. Hungry members are usually sick more often; this reduces household productivity in the short and over the longer term and also creates a demand for

11

additional medical care, which may go unmet because of limitations of time and money. The following two sections outline mechanisms through which hunger is transmitted intergenerationally.

Hunger among mothers and children

The malnutrition of pregnant women may lead to serious problems for their unborn children. Most dramatic is cretinism resulting from severe maternal iodine deficiency, discussed above. More commonly, children born to chronically undernourished women are likely to be small at birth. Low birth weight, which is associated with increased risk of mortality and with a range of health and developmental problems for survivors, may result either from premature delivery or from retarded intrauterine development. Maternal malnutrition is not the only cause of low birth weight but it is an important one. Women do not have to be malnourished during pregnancy to disadvantage their children; undernutrition during their own childhoods can cause growth stunting and influences the size of the child a woman can later bear. Maternal pelvic size is a strong determinant of neonatal survival and it is universally correlated with height in populations. The proportions of low birth-weight infants are much higher in populations identified as poorly nourished according to adult anthropometric indicators, ranging from lows of 4–6 per cent in many affluent countries to values of 25 per cent or greater in Pakistan, India, Bangladesh, and Laos (Grant 1990).

A mother's malnutrition may also limit her ability to breast-feed her infant. Quantity and quality of breastmilk are reduced in women who are severely undernourished, although lactation is often quite successful for mothers who are moderately malnourished. Especially under conditions of poverty, illiteracy, and poor sanitation, any threat to a mother's ability to breast-feed her baby is a threat to that baby's health and development. While affluent and well-educated mothers may safely choose to use commercial infant formula rather than breast-feed, the alternatives available to the very women whose own nutrition is likeliest to be marginal are less satisfactory and even life threatening. Alternative foods and breastmilk substitutes are lower in nutritional value and are likely to be contaminated. The additional immunological protection that breastmilk gives the infant is especially important under these conditions. Breastmilk substitutes are also relatively costly. They take resources that might otherwise be devoted to nutrition for other members of the household and therefore influence the health and nutrition of the entire household.

A young child's malnutrition influences not only its immediate health and well-being but also its later development. Where a child consumes less energy, it is less active. Avoidance of physical activity translates into a reduction in play and exploration and therefore impaired acquisition of communication, reasoning, and problem-solving skills. A child rendered apathetic, passive, and perhaps irritable by malnutrition invites less interaction with others. Cleland (1990) reviewed evidence that children receiving food supplements were more effective at communicating their needs than unsupplemented children. He also suggested that undernutrition of the whole family contributes to a more passive style of child care that causes health problems other than undernutrition to remain unaddressed.

In children, an additional adjustment to undernutrition is the slowing or cessation of physical growth. This is particularly damaging where the timing coincides with critical growth spurts, although growth shortfalls associated with hunger episodes usually can be made up if subsequent intake is sufficient to sustain catch-up growth as well as normal requirements. However, where hunger episodes alternate with periods of intake adequate only for normal needs, growth shortfalls may be permanent and cumulative. Early nutritional damage may be permanent in the absence of intensive remedial efforts.

Nutritional supplementation in impoverished conditions clearly has important benefits but its efficacy may also be limited. Longitudinal studies have shown that those receiving protein and energy supplementation at two years of age had better cognitive and occupational performance in adulthood (Chavez et al. 1995; Martorell 1995). In contrast, slum children receiving 1–4 years of nutritional supplementation and additional stimulation have been shown to lag behind those in more advantaged families (Lutter et al. 1989). Supplemented slum children outperformed others in their community, but the interventions were not enough to overcome their social disadvantage.

Special advantages for workers
Children's nutrient needs notwithstanding, the intrahousehold distribution of food has been shown sometimes to favour workers, who receive more food relative to need and more stable intakes despite seasonal fluctuations in household food availability (Gross and Under-

wood 1971; Van Esterik 1984). Patterns of discrimination that favour the most productive member(s) may be to the advantage even of those against whom they discriminate, if the protection of earning capacity protects the household's continued access to food and prevents further deterioration in nutritional status of most members.

Maternal nutrition may be especially important, since mothers usually manage the food, health, and care for all members. In addition, wages from maternal work have been shown to contribute directly to household food budgets and particularly the food available to children. Time diverted from meal preparation, however, can decrease dietary quality. Maternal work also may affect the intake of young children if they divert time from breast-feeding, special weaning-food preparation, or frequent feedings of toddlers (FAO 1987).

Food-poor households usually react to scarcity by seeking additional means of entitlement to food, including migratory wage labour, especially in urban areas. This reduces the number of consumers at home and adds migrant remittances to the household income stream. However, the irregularity of migrant remittances can contribute to inconsistent intake patterns. Also, reductions in labour available within the household have been known to cause shifts in household food production toward less labour-intensive crops, which are also often lower in nutritional value; non-staple crops such as vegetables may also be abandoned (Benería and Sen 1986; Tabatabai 1988). In sum, household strategies are designed to protect the nutrition and productivity of working members but demonstrate several disadvantages: they may further marginalize and undermine the nutritional status of dependents, they may not provide income security, and they may disrupt local subsistence production by diverting labour to other enterprises.

Effects of hunger beyond the household

Hunger cumulatively has effects beyond the household. Hunger and the threat of hunger are significant forces for social polarization. Strategies for avoiding hunger, misnamed "coping mechanisms," may permanently alter class and ethnic relations within communities and regions. For example, when other forms of entitlements fail, households are often forced to sell their productive assets to buy food. If many households in the same area are driven to employ the same strategy at the same time, all are likely to face depressed prices for their assets, from which the more secure households that are able to buy these assets improve their relative position. Actions to avoid hunger in the short run may jeopardize access to food in the long run and leave some permanently in food poverty, or at least more vulnerable to any further shocks. Whole populations may be forced to migrate in search of food, in the process disrupting development potential in a locality or region and encouraging political disorder and conflict.

The deleterious effects of hunger on individual work capacity also make it, in itself, a major obstacle to development. Households are not always able to nourish adequately even their most productive members. The low incomes and high energy expenditures usually associated with manual labour imply that those who need the most food can often afford the least.

Hunger also influences the next generation along multiple pathways. The biological changes brought about by hunger lead to altered behavioural and cognitive functioning, which in turn may condition social, economic, and political processes. Both economic development and family planning appear to be tied to effective schooling, but hunger directly affects children's ability to function in school and it increases incentives for families to keep their children out of school so that they can contribute to household income for food. The next generation, therefore, is less nutritionally prepared to improve its position.

The combination of low educational achievement and higher mortality rates among hungry families create a context in which limiting family size makes little economic sense. There are many other ways in which poverty contributes to population growth, but labour needs within households are particularly high where agricultural conditions are poor and where income diversification is an important means of assuring that *some* income will be available. High mortality decreases labour availability, and high childhood mortality dictates that sensible risk-minimizing strategies will include large numbers of births. It may seem counter-intuitive that families with few resources would not want to limit the number of ways those resources need to be divided, but this paradox can be best understood in this context of constant struggling for entitlement to food.

Organization of the volume

This book is organized to answer the question "who's hungry?" at three interrelated levels of social organization. Because the methodologies for estimating regional distribution of hunger differ from those used to estimate household and individual hunger, at each point we will also be asking the question "and how do we know?" We also highlight the limits of present knowledge since, without such understanding, there is a danger that unsupported assertions will be taken as factual and policy will be misinformed.

Our analysis is broad sweeping but it places emphasis on rural agricultural societies. This is justified because most of the world's hungry live in these societies.

Evaluations of hunger evidence begin in chapter 2, which specifically addresses basic measurement issues common to most estimations of hunger. Two contrasting strategies are presented: the first compares the diet actually consumed with that required and identifies cases in which the quantity or quality of that diet is inadequate; the second focuses on measurable outcomes of malnutrition. Each involves a range of problems, both in actual measurement and in defining the standard with which measured values must be compared.

Evidence as to the prevalence of food shortage is assembled and evaluated in chapter 3. Data on levels and trends in caloric availability at global, regional, and national levels are compared with estimates of requirements. Documentation of food shortages within more local areas is less abundant, but observed variations in the adequacy of food supplies across regions of the same country show that the cross-country picture is incomplete.

Food distribution is explored more comprehensively in chapter 4 on food poverty. Estimates of the numbers and percentages of people living in households that cannot afford to feed all of their members properly are presented by world region. These data are supplemented by country-level estimates of numbers in absolute poverty. Particularly vulnerable types of households are identified from comparisons of nutritional status across subgroups of national populations.

Chapter 5 analyses food deprivation and identifies which household members are at greatest risk. Comparisons of hunger along lines of age and gender are the major focus. Evidence from many diverse settings is reviewed, but particular attention is devoted to India, both because of rich data quality and because intra-household food allocation has been hypothesized to be particularly discriminatory in India.

Chapter 6 examines the central role of conflict as a determinant of food shortage, poverty, and deprivation. Although we do not dismiss the impact of fluctuations in the natural environment on food production, human responses to potential famine from droughts and floods are far more effective if such efforts are not limited by violent conflict. "Man-made disasters" and limitations on distribution of food, through both humanitarian and market channels, are also discussed in this chapter.

We must know who the hungry are in order to alleviate or prevent their hunger. Targets must be identifiable in order to design effective interventions. To address the underlying causes of hunger rather than merely attempt its amelioration, causes must be clearly understood. Our thinking with regard to the underlying causes of hunger can be refined by examining which people are most affected.

The concluding chapter discusses policy implications of the evidence reviewed, with particular attention to insights gained on the underlying causes of hunger. Multiple causes imply a wider choice of focus for intervention. The task of alleviating hunger may seem daunting, given the wide variety of its causes and the different levels of social organization on which they operate, but some of the underlying causes may be more susceptible to solutions than would be apparent from a less-complete understanding of who is hungry.

Works cited

Allen, L. H., A. K. Black, J. R. Backstrand, G. H. Pelto, R. D. Ely, E. Molina, and A. Chavez. 1991. "An Analytic Approach for Exploring the Importance of Dietary Quality Versus Quantity in the Growth of Mexican Children." *Food and Nutrition Bulletin* 13, No. 2: 95–104.

Barraclough, S. 1989. *An End to Hunger?* London: Zed Books.

Benería, Lourdes, and Gita Sen. 1986. "Accumulation, Reproduction, and Women's Role in Economic Development: Boserup Revisited." In: Eleanor Leacock, Helen I. Safa, and contributors, eds. *Women's Work: Development and the Division of Labor by Gender*. South Hadley, Massachusetts: Bergin & Garvey, pp. 141–157.

Brown, K. H. 1991. "The Importance of Dietary Quality Versus Quantity for Weanlings in Less Developed Countries: A Framework for Discussion." *Food and Nutrition Bulletin* 13, No. 2: 86–94.

Chavez, A., C. Martinez, and B. Soberanes. 1995. "The Effect of Malnutrition on Human Development: A 24 Year Study of Well-Nourished and Malnourished Children Living in a Poor Mexican Village." In: N. S. Scrimshaw, ed. *Community-Based Longitudinal Nutrition and Health Studies: Classic Examples from Guatemala, Haiti, and Mexico*. Boston: International Nutrition Foundation for Developing Countries, pp. 79–124.

Chen, Robert S. 1990. *Refugees and Hunger*. Providence, Rhode Island: Alan Shawn Feinstein World Hunger Program.

Cleland, John. 1990. "Maternal Education and Child Survival: Further Evidence and Explanations." In: John Caldwell, Sally Findley, Pat Caldwell, Gigi Santow,

Wendy Cosford, Jennifer Braid, and Daphne Broers-Freeman, eds. *What We Know About Health Transition: The Cultural, Social and Behavioral Determinants of Health*, Vol. I. Canberra: Health Transition Centre, The Australian National University, pp. 400–419.

Cousins, R. J., and J. M. Hempe. 1990. "Zinc." In: M. L. Brown, ed. *Present Knowledge in Nutrition*. Washington, D.C.: International Life Sciences Institute Nutrition Foundation, pp. 251–267.

FAO. 1987. "Women in African Food Production and Security." In: J. Price Gittinger, Joanne Leslie, and Caroline Hoisington, eds. *Food Policy: Integrating Supply, Distribution, and Consumption*. Baltimore: Johns Hopkins University Press, pp. 133–140.

Golden, B. E., and M. H. N. Golden. 1991. "Relationships Among Dietary Quality, Children's Appetites, Growth Stunting, and Efficiency of Growth in Poor Populations." *Food and Nutrition Bulletin* 13, No. 2: 105–109.

Grant, James P. 1990. *The State of the World's Children 1990*. New York: Oxford University Press for UNICEF.

———. 1995. *The State of the World's Children 1995*. New York: Oxford University Press for UNICEF.

Gross, Daniel R., and Barbara A. Underwood. 1971. "Technological Change and Caloric Costs: Sisal Agriculture in Northeastern Brazil." *American Anthropologist* 73, No. 3: 725–740.

Hamilton, Eva May Nunnelley, Eleanor Noss Whitney, and Frances Sienkiewicz Sizer. 1985. *Nutrition: Concepts and Controversies*. Third edition. St. Paul: West Publishing Company.

Hussey, G. D., and M. Klein. 1990. "A Randomized, Controlled Trial of Vitamin A in Children with Severe Measles." *New England Journal of Medicine* 323: 160–164.

Lutter, C. K., J. O. Moral, J.-P. Habicht, K. M. Rasmussen, D. S. Robson, S. G. Sellers, C. M. Super, and M. G. Herrera. 1989. "Nutritional Supplementation: Effects on Child Stunting Because of Diarrhea." *American Journal of Clinical Nutrition* 50: 1–8.

Martorell, Reynaldo. 1995. "Promoting Healthy Growth: Rationale and Benefits." In: Per Pinstrup-Andersen, David Pelletier, and Harold Alderman, eds. *Child Growth and Nutrition in Developing Countries*. Ithaca: Cornell University Press, pp. 15–31.

McGuire, Judith. 1991. "Quality Versus Quantity of Infant Diets: Translating Research Into Action." *Food and Nutrition Bulletin* 13, No. 2: 132–134.

Messer, E. 1996. "The Human Right to Food (1989–1994)." In: Ellen Messer and Peter Uvin, eds. *The Hunger Report: 1995*. Amsterdam: Gordon and Breach, pp. 65–82.

Millman, Sara R., Robert S. Chen, J. Emlen, V. Haarmann, Jeanne X. Kasperson, and Ellen Messer. 1991. *The Hunger Report: Update 1991*. Vol. HR-91-1. Providence, Rhode Island: Alan Shawn Feinstein World Hunger Program.

Newman, Lucile F., William Crossgrove, Robert W. Kates, Robley Mathews, and Sara Millman, eds. 1990. *Hunger in History: Food Shortage, Poverty and Deprivation*. Cambridge, Massachusetts: Basil Blackwell.

Oshaug, A., W. B. Eide, and A. Eide. 1994. "Human Rights: A Normative Basis for Food and Nutrition-Relevant Policies." *Food Policy* 19: 491–516.

Pelletier, David L. 1994. "The Potentiating Effects of Malnutrition on Child Mortality: Epidemiologic Evidence and Policy Implications." *Nutrition Reviews* 52, No. 12: 409–415.

Pollitt, E. 1991. "Effects of a Diet Deficient in Iron on the Growth and Development of Preschool and School-Age Children." *Food and Nutrition Bulletin* 13, No. 2: 110–118.

Ralte, Anne Lalsawmliani. 1996. "Progress in Overcoming Micronutrient Deficiencies: 1989–1994." In: Ellen Messer and Peter Uvin, eds. *The Hunger Report: 1995.* Amsterdam: Gordon and Breach, pp. 141–156.

Ramachandran, K. 1991. "'Reduced Mortality' with Vitamin A Supplementation." *NFI Bulletin (Bulletin of the Nutrition Foundation of India)* 12, No. 1: 6–7.

Rathmathullah, L., B. A. Underwood, R. D. Thulasiraj, R. C. Milton, K. Ramaswamy, R. Rathmathullah, and G. Babu. 1990. "Reduced Mortality Among Children in Southern India Receiving a Small Weekly Dose of Vitamin A." *New England Journal of Medicine* 323: 929–935.

Scrimshaw, Nevin S. 1990. "World Nutritional Problems." In: Lucile F. Newman, William Crossgrove, Robert W. Kates, Robley Mathews, and Sara Millman, eds. *Hunger in History: Food Shortage, Poverty, and Deprivation.* Cambridge, Massachusetts: Basil Blackwell, pp. 353–373.

Stanbury, J. B. 1991. "The Iodine Deficiency Disorders (IDD): Current Status." *Food and Nutrition Bulletin* 13, No. 4: 285–286.

Tabatabai, Hamid. 1988. "Agricultural Decline and Access to Food in Ghana." *International Labour Review* 127, No. 6: 703–734.

Tomkins, A., and F. Watson. 1989. *Malnutrition and Infection: A Review.* United Nations, Administrative Committee on Coordination, Subcommittee on Nutrition, ACC/SCN State-of-the-Art Series Discussion Paper No. 5. Geneva: World Health Organization.

Van Esterik, Penny. 1984. *Intra-Family Food Distribution: Its Relevance for Maternal and Child Nutrition.* Cornell University, Cornell Nutritional Surveillance Program Working Paper Series No. 31. Ithaca: Cornell University Press.

West, K. P. 1991. "Dietary Vitamin-A Deficiency: Effects on Growth, Infection, and Mortality." *Food and Nutrition Bulletin* 13, No. 2: 119–131.

2

Measuring hunger

Sara R. Millman and Laurie F. DeRose

Given the definition of hunger as consumption of a diet inadequate to sustain good health and normal activity, growth, and development, an ideal measure of hunger would involve a comparison between the diet actually consumed and that required for these purposes. In fact, one set of hunger indicators is based on this principle, focusing on the question of whether people are getting enough to eat. Practical implementation of the ideal, however, encounters significant difficulties both in measuring or estimating the diet and in defining the requirements against which it should be compared.

A second set of indicators focuses on outcomes of malnutrition. This approach has the advantage of identifying people whose intake is poor enough to have measurable consequences; it avoids the necessity of measuring either intake or need. But because some of the manifestations of hunger have other causes, it is not always clear that inadequate intake accounts for the outcome measured. To take an extreme example, death rates have been interpreted as aggregate indicators of hunger, and ratios of males to females in the surviving population as evidence of less adequate nutrition for one sex than the other. The possibility of other causes must also be kept in mind, even when using outcomes more directly related to food intake: anthropometric measurements may be influenced just as heavily by access to health care as by access to food.

An additional complication inherent in the use of outcomes of malnutrition as indicators of hunger is that these measurements must be compared with some standard of physical normality. This is most problematic with respect to growth. While the standards for what constitutes normal blood sugar levels are defined fairly precisely and uncontroversially, "normal growth" encompasses a wide range of alternatives: unhealthy growth patterns are more difficult to identify. This particular controversy will be explored in detail later in this chapter. For now, it is important to note that whether food intake or nutrition outcome is used as a measurement of hunger, standards are necessary.

Despite the great individual variability in intakes that would support good health and normal activity, cut-offs below which most would be functionally impaired can be defined. In measuring hunger and even in answering the more specific question of who is hungry, the use of standards allows us to identify types of individuals who are functionally impaired, even if some of those above the cut-offs also suffer from hunger and some below function normally. Chronic shortfalls in caloric availability in particular communities, or high proportions of underweight in particular sex and age groups, provide enough information to target interventions effectively. Nevertheless, we devote a great deal of attention to measurement issues in order to (1) identify the types of data that would be needed for future, more reliable, hunger estimates, (2) identify the biases inherent in some commonly used measurement techniques in order to inform interpretation of the statistics generated by them, and (3) explore the extent to which different indicators of hunger function interchangeably.

Input: Enough to eat?

To determine whether people are getting enough to eat requires the answers to two separate questions: what are people eating, and how much do they need? The former question is conceptually straightforward, but presents daunting data collection and estimation problems in practical terms. The latter compounds these problems. A diet that is adequate for some purposes is inadequate for others, since varying activity levels and patterns of growth can reconcile good health with a range of dietary intakes for the same individual. Thus, normative judgements as to desirable activity levels and growth patterns are implicit in any definition of dietary requirements. Uncertainties as to the range within which cost-free adaptation can occur and the factors underlying variation in requirements complicate the picture still further. Our review of hunger-estimation procedures that assess intake relative to need considers first the measurement of food availability and then the standards for need.

21

Food supplies

The discussion of estimates of food supply or dietary intake below is organized according to the three levels of social organization: these are the geographic region (in particular, the nation), the household, and the individual. Common approaches used to estimating food availability at each of these levels are described, with particular attention to measurement difficulties as well as sources of error and bias.

Food available to national populations

Estimates of national food supplies for most countries are maintained and regularly updated by the Food and Agriculture Organization (FAO) of the United Nations. These are based on food balance sheets, which involve detailed analyses of national food systems (see, e.g., FAO 1983, 1984). The accuracy of these accounts has been extensively questioned. The FAO estimates of per capita, per day food availability for national populations are an essential part of any attempt at either assessing hunger globally or exploring its variation across countries.

These estimates are obtained by first calculating the amounts of specific foods available for human consumption within the country. This is done by taking the sum of amounts produced, imported, or withdrawn from carry-over stocks and then subtracting amounts lost in processing or transport, used for purposes other than human food consumption (seed, feed for animals, industrial raw materials), exported, or stored for later use. Estimates of the nutrient content (calories, protein, and fat) per unit of each food are then multiplied by the amount of the food available to obtain estimates of the total amounts of each nutrient available from each foodstuff. These are summed across all foodstuffs to obtain total supplies of each specific nutrient. The final step is to divide national totals by the number of days in the period to which the supply data apply, and by the total number of people in the population. Thus, the results are commonly expressed as per day, per capita nutrient availability.

The data requirements of the food balance sheets are enormous. Precise values are often lacking for at least some of the necessary inputs. In other cases the situation may be one of no data at all for certain parameters, rather than of imprecise data. To the extent necessary, the blanks are filled in with approximations, assumptions, and informed guesswork. The resulting estimates, therefore, should not be viewed as unduly precise.

According to the FAO (FAO 1984), statistics on non-food utilization of food supplies are perhaps most widely problematic, while estimates of loss between harvest and household typically rest on reliable local expert opinions. And "...even the production and trade statistics on which the accuracy of food balance sheets depends most are, in many cases, subject to improvement..." (FAO 1984: ix) Uncertainties on withdrawals from and deposits to carry-over stocks are limited by preparing food balance sheet estimates as three-year averages.

The degree of imprecision may be greatest for exactly that set of countries in which the aggregate food supply is likeliest to be short, since general statistical systems are less well developed in poorer and less-industrialized countries than elsewhere and even population data may be lacking. In 20 of the 125 counties covered in detail in the World Bank's *World Development Report 1992* (World Bank 1992), the most recent census occurred in the 1970s or even earlier. Estimates of current populations extrapolated from past trends, or from old data that may have been inaccurate even when new, may be far from the truth. Nigeria's 1991 census, for example, counted a total of 88.5 million people, as compared with a UN estimate of 120.5 million people (APS 1992). Since dietary energy supply is divided by population to calculate per capita dietary energy supply, these alternative figures result in estimates that vary by 27.4 per cent. In this particular case, the food supply in Nigeria looks considerably more favourable when (presumably more accurate) data from the 1991 census are used instead of the older population estimates.

Food-production data may also be subject to extreme inaccuracies, especially in areas where much of the food produced is consumed directly by growers without ever entering the market. When such subsistence production occurs in remote regions it may be missed in national statistics. Even aerial surveys are likely to miss food production when it occurs as part of a system of shifting cultivation, with crops grown in small clearings in the jungle. Underestimation of available food is also particularly likely where uncultivated or lesser-known foods are commonly consumed. Some foods are omitted from food balance sheets entirely; in certain settings these may make up a significant portion of the total diet. Governments that tax and procure foods at below-market prices also present significant incentives for understatement of production by producers. These considerations will affect estimates of food production more in some areas than others, and therefore could bias the comparisons of relative food

23

availability using food balance sheets. Svedberg (1991) has argued that the FAO's food balance sheet approach significantly under-estimates food availability in sub-Saharan Africa relative to other regions. Despite their real shortcomings, however, food balance sheets provide the best information available as to national food supplies.

Household surveys

Surveys of representative samples of households are an alternative source for estimating national food supplies per capita. In addition, such surveys yield direct measures of household access to food. The FAO (1983) provides a useful comparison of several approaches.

Income/budget/expenditure surveys, with a broad focus on the economic situation of households, report amounts spent on food or the value of food consumed. Food quantities may be obtained as part of the process of estimating the value of food consumed, but are usually not shown in reports. This kind of survey omits food con-sumed outside the household and losses of food within the household; food gathered wild, received as a gift, and sometimes even produced by the household may also be omitted.

In contrast, food-consumption surveys focus more on amounts and nutrient composition of foods than on their economic value, and attempt to include food consumed away from home. Amounts may be ascertained by survey (recall), by consumption records maintained by the respondents, or by food weighing at meals (minus plate waste). Data collection (typically over a period of one to seven days for each household) is time-consuming and needs to be supervised for accu-racy. Not surprisingly, food-consumption surveys of samples large enough, and sufficiently dispersed geographically, to yield national statistics are largely unavailable. India is the only country that con-ducts such surveys routinely. Nevertheless, this strategy is used more frequently in local-area studies and yields valuable information.

Finally, items typical of either income/budget/expenditure surveys or food-consumption surveys may be incorporated in multiple-purpose surveys. The information about intake from these is less detailed than that from studies focused on food and nutrition, but they significantly contribute to what is known about household food availability. One example is the Living Standards Measurement Survey that the World Bank has sponsored in a number of developing countries.

Despite their advantages, survey data of the types described above are flawed, as indicators of either national food supplies or the distribution of food across households, by the short time span to which they typically apply. Since household food consumption and food expenditure do vary over time, a household's apparent food security may be very much affected by the duration and/or the timing of data collection. Even from one day to the next, household food consumption and expenditure are often highly variable. As recognized in some methodological treatises (e.g. National Research Council 1986), this short-term variation suggests that the shorter the period covered, the more frequently extreme values of calories per capita per day will be found. Therefore, shorter-term data collection will tend to find higher proportions of households at extremely low (or high) levels of dietary adequacy. The sensitivity of proportions observed at the lower extreme to measurement duration matters when measuring hunger. Although statistical adjustments are possible (National Research Council 1986), this problem often goes unrecognized and therefore uncorrected.

Temporal variations in food intake will have different effects on survey results, depending on whether they have a common cause that affects households similarly or whether the causes are more household specific. If patterns of temporal variation in household food security are unrelated across households (for example, job loss for some families in the absence of recession or widespread lay-offs), surveys taken at different times might find different sets, but similar proportions, of households unable to meet the needs of their members, and food consumption or expenditure totalled or averaged across households might be unaffected. If many households experience the same temporal pattern of food security, however, even the proportion of households falling below any specified cut-off and the total of consumption or expenditure across households may be very much affected by the timing of data collection.

In subsistence agriculture, for instance, a food-consumption survey taken just before harvest might well show a dire situation indeed, but one a few weeks later a situation of abundance. Neither snapshot reasonably characterizes the population's usual access to food. Even the per day, per capita caloric availability over a three-year period reflected in a food balance sheet would not capture this situation; the more compelling reality for understanding who is hungry may be exactly the wide swings between scarcity and abundance rather than the level to which these two extremes average. Only longitudinal data can capture this reality. Enough evidence exists to suggest that temporal variation is an important dimension of hunger in some settings,

25

but the research investment required to document such variation and its effect on the people who experience it leaves its details unexplored for most populations.

CONSUMPTION SURVEYS VERSUS SUPPLY METHODS. Overall, the consumption surveys versus supply methods of estimating national level food availability yield very different results. Comparing estimates of national per capita dietary energy supply based on income/budget/expenditure surveys and on food balance sheets, the FAO (1983) finds sizeable discrepancies. For developed countries, the survey results are consistently lower by hundreds of calories per day, at least partly owing to their omission of food consumed away from home. For developing countries, estimates from the two different sources also differ substantially, but the differences are smaller and not in a consistent direction. It is likely that the closer agreement of the two approaches for developing countries may reflect the fact that *both* surveys and food balance sheets underestimate food availability. Food balance sheets more accurately reflect availability in developed countries where most food is marketed than they do in developing countries. The more complete food balance sheet data for developed countries may eliminate a downward bias that would otherwise bring estimates into closer agreement with those based on income/budget/expenditure surveys.

In the FAO's assessment:

Annual food balance sheets tabulated regularly over a period of years will show the trend in the overall national food supply, disclose changes that may have taken place in the types of food consumed ... and reveal the extent to which the food supply of the country, as a whole, is adequate in relation to nutritional requirements ... (T)he food balance sheets ... while often far from satisfactory in the proper statistical sense, provide an approximate picture of the overall food situation in the countries which may be used for economic and nutritional studies, the preparation of development plans, and the formulation of related projects. (FAO 1984)

Despite their difficulties, the food balance sheets are the best information we have to quantify national food supplies for most countries of the world. Because they are collected yearly, using the same methodology, they can provide valuable information on the relative magnitude of year-to-year fluctuations in food availability (Atwood 1991). Although shifts in production (especially shifts to marketed crops) may change the proportion of production recorded by the

FAO even when total production remains unchanged, this type of change typically takes place over a number of years and is therefore unlikely to bias comparisons seriously between adjacent years.

Chapter 3 on food shortage in this volume draws on food balance sheets to assess the adequacy of national food supplies. They are also an essential input into global and regional estimates of numbers of people living in households that cannot afford the food their members need.

Food available to households
Even where the estimates of national per capita dietary energy supplies based on food balance sheets are quite accurate, they provide no clue about variable access to supply within nations. We know that some people go hungry, even in countries in which per capita total food supplies are far in excess of requirements, and that others are well fed, even in countries with too little food to meet the needs of their populations. We must have information on the distribution of food, not just the total amount available, in order to assess the prevalence of hunger. Surveys such as those discussed above provide one means of measuring variation across households in access to food.

With household-level food consumption or acquisition data, we can go beyond estimating the numbers of households, or of people in households, in food poverty. It is also possible to contrast the characteristics of households falling above or below some cut-off, or to compare access to food across different types of households. Both exercises help us to understand which households are hungry, not just how many. Household-level data also are indispensable for exploring associations between a household's food poverty status, health, education, and any other characteristics. Because nationally representative surveys gathering such information are scarce, our picture of household food poverty is necessarily incomplete. Many findings emerge from the literature on hunger and poverty; how widely these can be generalized is limited because there are so many settings for which the necessary data are not available.

A household's access to food is measured directly or estimated, and then compared with some standard of need to judge adequacy. The choice of cut-offs for minimally adequate food intake influences both the estimates of food poverty and the comparability across samples. The FAO and the World Bank now accept common standards, but the thresholds of undernutrition which they used even in the recent past were defined differently,[1] and both organizations regularly readjusted their methodologies (Uvin 1994). Therefore, comparative estimates of food poverty across time or across data sources both need to check which methodology was being used, to standardize reporting.

Household food surveys are used to help to define what income levels are necessary for households to enjoy different levels of access to food. Income levels measured in other data sets then can be translated into access to food, to estimate the adequacy of the diet for households for which no actual food data were gathered. The widely cited estimates of world hunger produced by the World Bank and the FAO estimate indirectly the distributions of household income and proportions of households falling below food adequacy. These are calculated country by country but published only for regions, in the expectation that errors in single-country estimates will tend to balance out in aggregation.

Single-country estimates of numbers of people living in households that cannot afford to feed their members have been published by the United Nations Development Programme (UNDP 1992) for many countries. These rely on national reports of numbers in absolute poverty, defined as inability to meet their needs for food and other basic necessities. In some instances, figures are given separately for rural and urban areas, permitting within-population comparison of food poverty along at least this one dimension. Operational definitions of absolute poverty are country specific; the situations captured by these country-specific operationalizations are not comparable across countries without further standardization to adjust for different underlying conditions and methodologies.

Food available to individuals within households

DIRECT MEASURES. Ultimately, we measure the hunger of individuals, whose access to food is regulated by intra-household allocation rules and processes. We know that some individuals go hungry in households enjoying food security, while certain individuals are well nourished even in households that are food insecure overall. Solid conclusions regarding intra-household allocation of food require direct measurement of individual food consumption. This form of data collection is even more demanding in terms of time and skill than the household food-consumption survey. In addition to ascertaining and recording kinds and quantities of foods prepared for, and left over after, every meal, the researcher must also keep track of which household member gets how much of each dish. Collecting this kind of data within households is never unobtrusive: even if it is not resented, it may result in some change in the actual consumption, especially if those observed believe that their ordinary behaviour is subject to disapproval. Understandably, few surveys collect individual food-consumption data for a large or nationally representative sample of households over an extended period of time.

Even when the effort is made, differences in the completeness of dietary information across household members can still confound comparisons. Some are likelier than others to do some of their eating outside the household (food may be provided on the job or at school, or may be purchased from street vendors) and such meals or snacks tend to be underreported. Children also "forage" – a practice that has led some anthropologists to insist that "child following" is the only reliable method to record their intakes (Wilson 1974; Laderman 1991).

One particularly vexing instance of such differential completeness of dietary data relates to the difficulty of measuring amounts of breast-milk consumed by small children. Many food-consumption studies report only on children over 12 months of age, but intake of children past infancy will be underestimated where breast-feeding extends into toddlerhood, as it commonly does in developing countries.

Breastmilk is often completely omitted from studies on individual food consumption; this is hardly surprising, given that some manuals on food-consumption study methodology (e.g. Cameron and Van Staveren 1988) give no recommendations for estimating its intake. Jelliffe and Jelliffe (1989) outlined considerable problems in measuring breastmilk intake and concluded that all of the methods in use produced inaccurate estimates. Nevertheless, even large-scale surveys can question women as to how frequently their children nursed, rather than just whether they nursed. More labour-intensive surveys can observe women going about their daily tasks and count breast-feeding bouts over a full 24 hours.[2] These methods could provide a better indication of how important breastmilk is in the diet of children in different cultures. An indication – rather than a precise measurement – is all that is going to be available from dietary-survey data. More accurate methods, such as isotope dilution of labelled water, are too costly to be used in large-scale surveys.

The frequent omission of breastmilk from food-consumption data may qualify the common finding that the youngest are worst fed. While there are undoubtedly times and places in which children do

29

receive less than a fair share of household food supplies, the downwards bias on estimates of food consumption for the youngest, resulting from omission of mother's milk, may both exaggerate such a pattern where it exists and create one where it does not.

INDIRECT MEASURES. The difficulty of collecting data on individual food consumption has led some researchers to use less-direct measures. For example, the order in which different household members are served at meals often is interpreted as an indicator of relative access to the common food supply, and the conclusion is drawn that those served last receive less than a fair share (e.g. den Hartog 1973; Katona-Apte 1975; Maher 1981; Papanek 1990).

Reports that certain foods are normatively forbidden to, or reserved for, people in particular age, gender, or status categories provide a second set of indicators of within-household differences in access to food and the relative adequacy of diets. These observations suggest differences in dietary adequacy within a household. However, without further measurement of actual intakes compared with some nutritional standard they are not conclusive. More effort has to be made to validate these kinds of intra-household consumption indicators; where individual food-consumption data are available, it would be useful to explore the extent to which inferences that could be drawn from eating order and other aspects of dietary tradition are borne out.

Nutritional requirements

Measures of food supply available to national populations, accessible to households, or consumed by individuals always must be compared with amounts required, in order to permit any conclusion as to adequacy. Our discussion of nutritional requirements, that here focuses on energy, covers the same three levels of social organization as the preceding discussion of food availability; however, because the requirements for larger aggregations of people are conceptually based on the sum of individual requirements, we proceed from the individual, to the household, to the population.

Individual requirements
According to the United Nations:

The energy requirement of an individual is the level of energy intake from food that will balance energy expenditure when the individual has a body size and composition, and level of physical activity, consistent with long-term good health; and that will allow for the maintenance of economically necessary and socially desirable physical activity. In children and pregnant or lactating women, the energy requirement includes the energy needs associated with the deposition of tissue or the secretion of milk at rates consistent with good health. (WHO 1985: 12)

These requirements vary across individuals and within individuals over time. They are influenced by gender, body size, physical activity level, age, reproductive status, and disease. In addition, cross-population variation unexplained by these factors appears to reflect some influence of climate as well as other factors, such as dietary composition. But individuals who appear comparable on all these dimensions and who are in energy balance, as indicated by absence of weight loss or gain, still vary widely in their caloric intake. Consequently, accurate determination of an individual's caloric requirements would necessitate very intensive data collection under laboratory conditions. This is clearly infeasible on any large scale. Thus, studies of individual dietary adequacy most commonly compare actual intake with expected or average per capita requirements for persons similarly classified on the same background variables.

The most contentious and difficult aspect of caloric requirements relates to adaptations to a constrained diet. Desirable patterns of growth for children and desirable patterns of physical activity at all ages are an important part of this controversy. Some analysts (e.g. Sukhatme 1988) have argued that intake and expenditure of dietary energy function as a self-regulating homoeostatic system in which the efficiency of energy use is increased as intake decreases and decreased as intake increases. The argument is a rather technical one, but its real-world implications are far from trivial. It has been taken as demonstrating "cost-free" adaptation to low intake – the possibility of maintaining not only energy balance and health but even usual activity levels on severely restricted consumption.[3]

Others have responded (see, e.g., Scrimshaw and Young 1989; Waterlow 1989) that adaptation to low intakes does not occur without undesirable limitation of physical activity. A *proportion* of the reduction in energy use that occurs as a result of reduced intake is apparently innocuous: weight loss itself causes some decline in caloric requirements, and less energy is used in digestion, absorption, and storage of nutrients when less food is consumed. However, the major mechanisms for reduced energy expenditure are behavioural. Therefore, most nutritionists do not view the adaptation to low intakes as cost free.

Although controversial, the concept of cost-free adaptation may well underlie decisions by some major nutrition-monitoring organizations (e.g. FAO 1977, 1985; NNMB 1981) to define cut-offs for undesirably low caloric intake at levels two standard deviations below average requirements. Setting such low cut-offs for minimal intake guarantees that the prevalence of hunger will not be overestimated. But unless the people with the lowest intakes also have the lowest requirements, it also guarantees that a high proportion of cases of genuinely inadequate intake will go unrecognized.

The controversy about the degree of adaptation to nutritional stress is also a policy debate about resource allocation. Few would argue that adaptation to extreme deprivation could be cost free, but those who interpret adaptation to lower levels of nutritional stress as cost free favour allocating resources to more narrowly focused nutritional programmes that would benefit only those in extreme need. If their premise is correct, this would reduce expenditure while increasing effectiveness. Those who have higher estimates of the costs of more moderate deprivation emphasize the needs of marginally nourished people. Their arguments tend to focus on the difficulty of emerging from poverty when productivity is limited by intake (e.g. Dasgupta and Ray 1990). If this is the case, government expenditure on broader nutrition programmes represents a better long-term policy choice, since it will improve both national productivity and national income distribution.

Household requirements
To estimate requirements for aggregations of individuals, whether these be households or national populations, it is necessary to consider what kinds of individuals make them up. Households are commonly defined – even outside the literature on hunger – as groups of individuals who share cooking facilities. Some individuals have regular access to food in more than one household (e.g. polygynous men whose wives do not cook together), and this complicates the estimation of household need.

Household need is determined by the number of members as well as their age, gender, and other determinants of individual need listed above. For households, caloric requirements are often estimated as the product of household size and national average per capita requirements. The implicit assumption is that each household's com-

Table 2.1 **Percentage of households in food poverty by definition of household caloric requirements, Indonesia, 1980**

		Household requirements defined by product of household size and national per capita requirement		
		Households below cut-off	Households above cut-off	Total
Household require-ments defined as sum of individual requirements	Households below cut-off	47.26	5.62	52.88
	Households above cut-off	5.29	41.83	47.12
	Total	52.55	47.45	100.00

Source: Data from the Indonesian National Socio-Economic Survey of 1980; tabulation by Mark M. Pitt.

position mirrors that of the nation as a whole. In fact, of course, households differ in their composition: the nutritional needs of a woman living with three children under five differ substantially from those of a childless couple living with two of the husband's brothers. Although estimates of household requirements reflecting each house-hold's own composition are preferable in principle, detailed analysis of Indonesian data (see table 2.1) suggest that the additional ana-lytical effort involved makes little difference to the proportions of households estimated to consume less than they need. Approximately equal numbers of households are misclassified in each direction by relying on national average per capita requirements. Thus, although misclassification does occur for many households, aggregate results are virtually unaffected, at least for this population.

Caloric consumption requirements for households are the sum of the requirements of their individual members. However, if require-ments are to be compared with measures of food supplies available to a household, rather than with those actually eaten within it, some allowance should be made for loss or wastage of food within the household. Such losses occur, for example, owing to spoilage, to infestation by insects or other pests, to losses in preparation, or to "plate waste" – leftovers discarded. While plate waste may be low in situations of scarcity, poor storage facilities make it difficult to avoid other forms of food loss within the household. More-affluent house-holds may have the storage facilities needed to minimize spoilage but are less likely to make sure every bit of edible food is consumed.

Thus, for different reasons, some loss of food is expected in both poorer and wealthier households.

National requirements

Determining caloric need for national populations is somewhat less complicated, because the fluidity of boundaries between households is not an issue and the gender and age composition of national populations is generally well known. Estimates of average per capita caloric requirements for national populations incorporate information on typical body sizes and physical activity levels, as well as age and sex composition, and may also allow for effects of childhood disease and desired growth patterns for children.

Several sets of average per capita caloric-requirements estimates for national populations have been published by various organizations and applied widely. Unfortunately, requirements estimates for the same population may vary substantially. More unfortunately still, some statistical compendia present caloric availability data only as a proportion of requirements, without specifying what standards for requirements are being used. Thus, the potential for confusion and contradiction is substantial. The remainder of this section briefly reviews some of the reasons for the differences in sets of requirements estimates.

Estimates of national average per capita caloric requirements produced by the FAO were published in the *Fourth World Food Survey* (FAO 1977) and have been used since in preparation of several kinds of national-level estimates of hunger. FAO publications from 1990 (e.g. FAO 1990a, 1990b, 1990c), however, show a different set of caloric-requirements estimates, in most cases substantially lower than the old ones.

The difference between these sets of estimates – a median decrease of 280 calories per day – was enough to result in drastically different pictures of world hunger. For example, the total 1987 population of countries with per capita caloric availability below requirements was 1,603 million relative to the old requirements, but 152 million relative to the new ones (Millman and Chen 1991). The difference turns out to be attributable to two main factors. First, the new estimates incorporate new (and presumably more accurate) data on body sizes of national populations. In most cases, this new information contributed to a reduction in requirements estimates. Second, and more significant, the reduced FAO caloric-requirements estimates eliminate an allowance for food losses within the household or retail establishment. The FAO's food balance sheets do account for losses of food prior to harvest and during food storage, processing, and delivery to retail establishments, but they no longer allow for losses within households or institutions. In the past, their caloric requirements estimates were inflated by 10 per cent to allow for such losses.

Not accounting for food loss within households amounts to making the unrealistic assumption that its value is zero. Some allowance would seem essential in assessing the adequacy of supplies of food available to households or to national populations. Comparisons of hunger prevalence at different points in time should not be made without attention to the standards applied, or misleading conclusions as to trend may result. Comparisons made using data published since 1992 are less problematic because the FAO and the World Bank have adopted a common methodology for producing their estimates.

The balance of food supply and requirements

At each level of social organization that we consider, conclusions about hunger are seriously affected by the measurement issues raised in this chapter. We draw attention to the methodological difficulties in the study of hunger, not to create pessimism about our ability to measure hunger but to inform comparisons between results derived from different practices. Assessments of food shortage may under-estimate production and underestimate waste, but, as we have emphasized, the most commonly used methods are likely to yield re-liable data about trends in food security. Employing even faulty methodologies consistently gives us a picture of how the balance of food supply and requirements is changing, and can even help identify what factors are influencing the changes.

Assessments of food poverty may be flawed by lack of attention to household composition or the changeable nature of household boundaries, but we have shown that these issues are unlikely to affect estimated levels of food poverty profoundly. In chapter 5 we will address how these and other issues affect our understanding of *which* households are in food poverty.

Comparisons across countries, of the extent of food poverty or the determinants of food poverty, may be flawed or reach varying con-clusions if they fail to account for different types of data and defi-nitions employed within countries. Studies that measure household food availability by documenting consumption cannot be directly compared with those that estimate food poverty on the basis of low income. But important insights into the determinants of hunger can result from comparing methodologies and outcomes in a single setting that can then guide additional research. If household income seems to be adequate and household food consumption is unacceptably low, the determinants of spending patterns then deserve more attention than the determinants of income. If certain households seem to do a better job than others, of balancing intake with requirements despite income constraints, then focusing on nutritional strategies and sources of food and income in those households might be productive.

Assessments of food deprivation based on intake must be careful to consider individual requirements when drawing conclusions, especially where judgements of discrimination leading to inadequate intake are involved. Some studies of intra-household food allocation have concluded that women and children received less than their fair share because they consumed fewer calories per day than others. If everybody had the same caloric requirements, differences in consumption could, indeed, be interpreted as showing patterns of advantage and disadvantage. But caloric requirements do vary and, typically, are lower for women and children than for others. To reach meaningful conclusions on adequacy or equity, dietary comparisons must examine individual intake relative to individual need. This can be done by dividing each household member's consumption by the corresponding estimate of requirements and comparing the results, often referred to as indices of dietary adequacy or caloric adequacy, which can be interpreted to show patterns of discrimination or equity. Only where the ratio of consumption to requirements is lower for women than for men, and for children than their elders, can we then conclude that women and children are at a disadvantage in the intra-household allocation of food. The additional complication of gender bias built into standards is discussed further in the section on choice of standards.

Another set of studies bases conclusions about discriminatory allocation of food within the household on the observation that certain household members are eating less than they need, without demonstrating that others are doing any better. In these instances, we usually have solid evidence of inadequate diets for those identified as victims. Again, however, a comparison with the situation of others is necessary to support a conclusion of relative disadvantage: other household members may be equally underfed, and, if so, our interpretation of the situation should be quite different from that if we find that others in the same household consume a more adequate diet. If all are underfed, the household is clearly in food poverty and food deprivation is being experienced by all its members. If only some are food deprived, this may or may not result from food poverty.

Output: Nutritional outcomes

We now turn our attention to the second set of hunger indicators, those based on measuring outcomes of malnutrition. This section focuses almost exclusively on anthropometric measurements, both because they are widely used and because they are the subject of considerable controversy. However, it is important to note that micronutrient deficiencies are also important because of their significant functional consequences, described in the introductory chapter, and also because they can signal other problems in dietary adequacy. Correctly diagnosing clinical signs of micronutrient deficiency requires well-trained staff and more extensive data: making comparisons between populations is only now becoming possible. If means of identifying mild-to-moderate deficiencies become available, these could provide increasingly important tools for measuring hunger.

Nutritional status is most commonly measured, especially in young children, by anthropometry – measurement of dimensions of physical size, such as height or weight, and comparison with distributions of the same measurement in a presumably healthy and well-nourished reference population. Children whose weight falls below the range of normal variation for children of the same age observed in a reference population are identified as underweight. Underweight may reflect small stature, excessive thinness, or both. These two dimensions are differentiated in two more refined anthropometric measures – weight for height and height for age. If the child's weight falls below the range of normal variation for children of the same height, it is considered wasted. If its height falls below the range of normal variation for children of the same age, it is considered stunted. Wasting is generally interpreted as an indicator of acute malnutrition – a current or recent crisis involving extreme weight loss. Stunting, in contrast, indicates early malnutrition. Either a past episode (or episodes) of acute malnutrition, or a routinely limited diet over an extended period, has resulted in growth impairment, even though current nutrition may be adequate.

Anthropometry is used to assess adults as well as young children, but this is done less widely. Shortness, although it may be nutritionally caused, provides clues only to the individual's experience during childhood, so that adult heights are uninformative regarding current or recent nutrition. Thinness, however, implies current undernutrition for adults as it does for children. Thus, weight for height is relevant across the range of ages, as are such other measures of fatness as mid-upper arm circumference (MUAC), skinfolds, or the body mass index. Although it is thus possible to measure people of all ages using the same anthropometric indicators, this rarely occurs in practice. As a result, evaluation of commonly stated conclusions regarding age patterns of variation in nutritional status is often quite difficult.

Anthropometry as an indicator of individual malnutrition

Anthropometry alone is not sufficient to diagnose nutritional problems in individuals, although it identifies children whose situation should be examined further in making such a diagnosis.[4] If the lower bounds of normal variation were set so low as to exclude all cases of healthy small size, much actual malnutrition would not register. In order to obtain a reasonable degree of sensitivity, cut-offs are set high enough that a small proportion of individuals fall below them, despite good health and adequate nutrition. At the same time, some who are naturally larger may fall above the cut-offs, even when they are, in fact, malnourished.

The lower limit of the range of normal variation in anthropometry has been variously operationalized. One common practice has been to define a cut-off at some set percentage of the median from the reference population. For weight for age, 80 per cent has been the most widely used cut-off, but milder or more severe underweight has been defined in terms of higher or lower percentage cut-off points. For other anthropometric measures, different percentage cut-off points have been identified. Recent work has more consistently used a cut-off two standard deviations below the mean of the reference population. Using standard deviations is preferred to using percentage cut-offs because comparability across measures and for the same measure at different ages is not compromised by greater or lesser variability. Roughly 3 per cent of healthy children will be more than two standard deviations below the mean of a healthy reference population, but most children this small are correctly identified as being at nutritional risk. Those more than two standard deviations below the mean are usually identified as moderately malnourished, while those falling three standard deviations or more below the mean are severely malnourished. Some researchers have suggested using a cut-off of one standard deviation in order to target nutritional supplementation programmes to those at risk of undernutrition (see comments in Popkin 1994). While it is desirable to enhance marginal diets of children who are showing no clinical signs of growth faltering, it is preferable to target children at greater risk, if resources are limited. It is worth repeating that none of these cut-off points has any necessary functional significance, despite their utility in helping to identify hungry individuals.

Meaningful individual diagnosis involves repeated measurement over time. Repeated measurement allows a child's growth trajectory to be compared with that of normal growth, rather than simply relying on a one-time measurement relative to a cut-off point. The repeated measurement process is referred to as "growth monitoring" and can be used to determine if small children are growing normally; it can also identify larger children whose growth has become compromised, even before their size drops below some cut-off. Weight loss, as opposed to unusually low weight, is a more reliable indicator of nutritional crisis. Similarly, a period during which no increase in height occurs tells us more than does a one-point observation of unusual shortness, which might have resulted either from such a crisis (or repeated crises) at any time up to the present or from a pattern of uninterrupted slow growth. Growth monitoring has been promoted as part of the UNICEF/WHO "GOBI" (growth monitoring, oral rehydration therapy, breast-feeding, and immunizations) initiative for child survival. Its utility in this context is in alerting the mother and the health practitioner to developmental problems at an earlier stage, and thus encouraging intervention before much damage has occurred.

Anthropometry as an indicator of malnourished groups

Cross-sectional anthropometric measures are less ambiguous indicators of nutritional problems for groups than they are for individuals. While the lesser growth potential of some individuals may cause them to register as underweight, wasted, or stunted, even when they are in good health and well fed, such individuals will be rare. If the proportion of individuals so identified in any group is high, we can be more sure that malnutrition is a significant problem for this group than that each individual identified is necessarily malnourished.

This assumes, however, that the reference population defining the range of normal variation is appropriate – that the target population would, in fact, show the same distributions of weights for age, weights for height, and heights for age if it, too, were healthy and well nourished. The most commonly used growth standards for international research are US based, and there is real controversy as to whether US growth standards are necessarily applicable everywhere. It has been argued that, in populations facing nutritional constraint over the long term, small size may, in fact, represent a healthy adaptation rather than indicating a problem (see review in Osmani 1992). Since nutritional requirements are, in part, a function of body size, stunted growth helps keep requirements low for individuals and populations and may permit good health and normal functioning at intake levels that would be too low if size were larger.

This controversy has clear implications for measuring hunger. If populations vary with respect to their proportion of *healthy* individuals whose anthropometric measurements fall far below the mean of the reference population, using any absolute cut-off would bias comparisons of hunger prevalence between populations. Such an argument, in fact, makes cross-country comparisons of hunger virtually impossible: any variation in achieved stature or even in caloric intake could be explained as adaptation rather than evidence of hunger. Although we argue that cross-country comparisons are both desirable and useful, we also consider the arguments against our position very carefully. The remainder of this section reviews three major arguments for why US-based growth standards might be inappropriate. We then address the question of how much difference the choice of a growth standard makes to our understanding of who is hungry.

Natural selection for small body size?
"Healthy adaptation" to nutritional constraint may occur at the population – rather than the individual – level. Evolutionary pressures may have favoured small size in populations facing a very constrained diet. This variant of the "small but healthy" argument suggests that genetically determined potential size is actually less in those populations (such as most of South Asia) where average body size is small by Western standards.

However, numerous studies have demonstrated that élite groups in such populations, less constrained in terms of both diet and health care, show growth patterns (at least in early childhood) that are quite similar to those reflected in the US-based growth standards. Genetic potential for these élite groups within populations of small average size does not appear strikingly less than for their Western counterparts. Marked increases in stature from one generation to the next are commonly observed when individuals from populations of small average stature migrate into countries with larger average stature. These increases, which are generally associated with changes in the diet and health, are difficult to reconcile with the notion that small statures in the areas of origin result from genetically determined limited growth potential. Similar very rapid increases in average stature within populations undergoing dietary enrichment (Japan, China), often associated with modernization or increasing affluence, also suggest that growth potential is comparable in populations between which actual attained body sizes vary widely.

Individual adaptation to nutritional constraint?
Even if the small body sizes observed in nutritionally constrained populations are not genetically determined, an adaptive mechanism rooted in individual experience remains a possibility. We know both that nutritional constraint during childhood is a cause of permanently small body size and that small body size in turn reduces lifetime nutritional requirements. The question then becomes, at what cost is this lifelong economy won? We can separate the answer to this question into two parts – costs of being, and of becoming, small.

To be small in stature means, *ceteris paribus*, to be less powerful physically than if one were taller. Since the poorest, who are likeliest to suffer growth impairment, are also probably likelier than others to have to earn their living through hard physical labour, this cost may be significant in terms of lost productivity and earnings. In contrast, small size itself may not be a problem for those whose work is mental rather than physical.

Small mothers are also at higher relative risk of bearing low birth-weight babies. The physical mechanisms through which maternal stunting is linked to birth weight are not completely understood. It has also not been conclusively demonstrated that stunting in the absence of other nutritional problems (e.g. underweight, anaemia) or deprivation during pregnancy adversely affects birth weight (Osmani 1992). Nevertheless, the correlation between maternal height and birth weight is strong across a large number of populations. Even if maternal stunting serves only as a proxy for the conditions that place children at high risk, it is still a useful indicator of who is likely to be hungry.

Some nutritionists (e.g. Beaton 1989) argue that, while there is nothing wrong with *being* small, the process of *becoming* small is

41

damaging. Increased risks of morbidity and mortality are among the major concerns. As Martorell (1995) argued:

Although growth retardation does not *cause* depressed immunocompetence, the factors that cause growth faltering, such as infection and inadequate intakes of specific nutrients, also result in immunodepression ... children may get infected for reasons largely determined by their environment, but, once they are infected, the course of the infection will be influenced strongly by nutritional status, reflected by the degree of growth retardation.

Even if increased risks of morbidity and mortality could be ruled out, the advantages of small size should not be counted as cost free if the constraints resulting in small size also cause significant functional impairment. Associations of growth impairment with poor intellectual and social development are well documented, and there are plausible mechanisms by which the same processes of malnutrition that cause impaired growth may also cause developmental impairments.

The small size associated with nutritional constraint has often been equated with increased risks of mortality – so strongly so, in the minds of some, that the infant mortality rate has been suggested as "one of the best tools available for measuring the extent of hunger in a society" (THP 1983), and growth has been called "the most important single indicator of health" for a child (Grant 1990). Others (Mosley and Chen 1984) have recommended that analysts combine growth impairment and mortality into a single variable, with survivors classified according to the Gomez scale of weight for age (relative to the median from an applicable growth chart, 89–75 per cent is grade I malnutrition, 74–60 per cent is grade II, less than 60 per cent is grade III) and then creating a fourth (grade IV) category for non-survivors. An assumption implicit in each of these suggestions is not only that underweight is strongly associated with elevated risks of mortality but also that the form of this relationship is relatively invariant.

There is certainly reason to expect malnutrition to increase risks of morbidity and mortality, as discussed in chapter 1. Malnutrition does reduce resistance to some infectious diseases, with different aspects of the immune system affected by deficiencies of varying degree with respect to specific nutrients. Many studies demonstrate cross-sectional associations between malnutrition and morbidity (for a useful review, see Tomkins and Watson 1989) or mortality (Puffer and Serrano 1973). In cross-sectional studies, however, effects of illness on nutritional status confound the effect of nutritional status on illness, and effects of nutritional status itself on survival chances are confused with effects of illness on both. Longitudinal research linking anthropometry to subsequent morbidity or mortality is relatively scarce.[5] When this is done, reverse causation can be ruled out, although surrounding circumstances (such as crowding or poor sanitation) that cause frequent illness could be responsible for both malnutrition and other adverse outcomes. At the extremes of malnutrition, there is no doubt that a range of adverse outcomes become increasingly likely.

However, some poor areas considered to have extraordinarily low infant and child mortality for their level of economic development (e.g. Sri Lanka, the state of Kerala in India) also have very high prevalences of underweight in small children. In contrast, some countries with the very highest rates of mortality in infancy and early childhood (including much of sub-Saharan Africa) exhibit relatively moderate prevalences of underweight. Since disease is a major cause of both malnutrition and death, a positive association between aggregate indicators of underweight and mortality would be expected even if malnutrition did nothing to increase risks of death. Deviations from the expected pattern at the aggregate level require further investigation. Further research might show that factors such as access to health care or maternal education mediate the relationship between body size and mortality; small stature may be a significant but surmountable mortality risk factor. If other variables, in fact, play an important mediating role in the body size/survival relationship, high proportions of underweight, wasting, or stunting might accurately reflect important variations in nutritional adequacy rather than simply measurement problems.

In summary, two additional conclusions about the desirability of individual adaptation to low food availability deserve emphasis. First, as outlined in chapter 1, limitations on physical activity due to lethargy during childhood have both physical and intellectual consequences. Second, stronger manual labourers may be able to earn more than enough to compensate for the increased caloric needs associated with their larger size. Although it seems likely that individual adaptation to low intake occurs regularly, anthropometric measurements are still useful hunger indicators.

Distinctive growth patterns of breast-fed and formula-fed infants
Applying US-based anthropometric standards to infants is another controversial area, since the US standard reflects the experience of mostly formula-fed infants who were supplemented with solid food

fairly early in life (Ahn and MacLean 1980). Furthermore, at the time the data for the standards were collected, more nutrient-dense infant formulas were used than is now the case. Under circumstances where adequate amounts of formula can be given and hygiene maintained, the use of modern infant formula leads to more rapid weight gain, at least after the first few months, than does breast-feeding (Ritchie and Naismith 1975; Stuff and Nichols 1989). This divergence in growth trajectories has been conventionally interpreted as showing that un-supplemented breastmilk is sufficient only for the infant's first four to six months, the period before the growth paths diverge. It is therefore recommended that other foods should be added to the infant's diet even if breast-feeding continues beyond the first four or six months (see, e.g., Underwood and Hofvander 1982).

Nevertheless, a number of researchers have argued that the standard reflects a less-than-optimal growth pattern (Ahn and MacLean 1980; Huffman 1991; Whitehead and Paul 1984). Whitehead and Paul argued that there was no reason for concern when children fall behind standards based on "inappropriately constituted and adminis-tered formulae." This conclusion seems especially appropriate in view of medical evidence that breast-fed children who show growth faltering relative to the standard can be shown to be just as healthy or healthier, according to other measures. They have fewer respiratory infections and less incidence of diarrhoea (Chandra 1982), and their energy requirements are lower because of their smaller body size, lower heart rates, and lower metabolic rates – not because of lower levels of physical activity (Garza and Butte 1990). They are also un-likely to be undernourished since their caloric intakes do not increase when their diets are supplemented with solids (Garza and Butte 1990; Stuff and Nichols 1989).

Such findings lead researchers to question whether all infants *ought* to follow the growth patterns that can be achieved with infant for-mula. If more rapid growth is not advantageous, application of stan-dards based on the experience of bottle-fed infants may overstate the prevalence of underweight in populations where most children are breast-fed and may also lead to a perception that supplementation is needed at ages at which breastmilk still fully meets the infant's needs. Where surrounding conditions make it difficult to maintain good hygiene, unnecessarily early introduction of supplementary foods that are likely to be contaminated may increase rather than lessen risks of malnutrition.

Growth standards still need to be developed that reflect the experience of exclusively breast-fed children and children receiving non-formula supplements. Until that time, cross-country comparisons using anthropometric measurements should be interpreted with special caution for the youngest children. The main difference in growth patterns between breast-fed and formula-fed children is faster weight gain in the formula-fed group (Garza and Butte 1990), and the greatest difference in weight gain is associated specifically with formula feeding, not other methods of artificial feeding. Therefore, comparisons of stunting (height for age) are less likely to be affected by use of the US-based standards than are comparisons of underweight. The greatest caution needs to be applied when comparing weight gain in populations where breast-feeding is common versus those where commercial infant formula is widely used.

How much difference does choice of growth standard make?

As the discussion above suggests, selection of an appropriate reference standard for anthropometric measurements is a contentious issue. For international purposes, use of the National Center for Health Statistics (NCHS) standard (based on the experience of children in the United States) has been recommended by the World Health Organization and is now widely accepted. Some countries, however, have chosen to develop and use local standards instead. Typical growth patterns do vary across populations, and the issue is which deviations ought to be viewed as problematic and avoidable.

Implications of this choice for our understanding of hunger are not trivial (Millman et al. 1991). Different anthropometric standards can yield very different estimates of the prevalence of malnutrition in the same population. For India, for example, estimates of the prevalence of underweight among children based on the NCHS or the local (Hyderabad) standard differ by 25.7 percentage points for 1989 (NNMB 1989). If local growth standards reflect the experience of less-than-healthy adaptation, their use will define real nutritional problems out of existence (Messer 1986).

Less obvious, but equally problematic, is that the choice of standard can also affect the analyst's understanding of which groups within a population are worse off. In particular, the contrast between the prevalence of malnutrition observed for males and females can be very much affected by the standard employed. Within each standard, sep-

Table 2.2 **Median weights (kg) for age and sex compared between Hyderabad and NCHS standards**

Age (years)	Boys			Girls		
	Hyderabad	NCHS	Ratio	Hyderabad	NCHS	Ratio
1+	10.50	11.5	0.91	9.80	10.8	0.91
2+	12.50	13.5	0.93	11.30	13.0	0.87
3+	14.75	15.7	0.94	13.30	15.1	0.88
4+	17.25	17.7	0.97	15.65	16.8	0.93

Source: for the Hyderabad standard, NNMB (1989); for the NCHS standard, Dibley et al. (1987).

arate reference values are defined for males and females, a complication necessary to capture typical healthy growth patterns for boys and girls. Any standard embodies the pattern of gender contrast that typifies the population on which it is based. A standard based on a population in which treatment of boys and girls differs in nutritionally consequential ways essentially defines the resulting differentiation of developmental paths as the norm. For example, the Hyderabad standard used in India, which is based on the experience of a population of urban middle-class children in southern India, incorporates a pattern of male advantage as compared with the US-based and internationally used NCHS standard. Table 2.2 contrasts median weights by age and sex in the two standards. While the Hyderabad standard in general defines lower weights as normal than does the NCHS one, the point here is that the downward shift in median weight associated with the use of the Hyderabad standard is greater for females than for males.

Distributions of weight for age that imply the same prevalence of malnutrition for boys and for girls as compared with the NCHS standard would inevitably show higher rates of malnutrition for boys than for girls if the Hyderabad standard were employed. Conversely, a situation that appears to be one of gender equality in malnutrition relative to the Hyderabad standard would show a female disadvantage if the presumably non-gender-biased NCHS standard were employed.

Table 2.3 shows the sharply different patterns of gender contrast that are observed when the same situation is viewed through the lens of one or the other weight-for-age standard. Tabulations of 1989 data for seven states of India (NNMB 1989) based on the Hyderabad

Table 2.3 **Gender comparisons: Underweight Indian children according to the Hyderabad and NCHS standards, 1989**

Standard	Percentage of boys underweight	Percentage of girls underweight	Female advantage (boys – girls)
NCHS	61.9	60.0	1.9
Hyderabad	42.5	28.0	14.5

Source: NNMB (1989).

standard show an apparent nutritional advantage for girls, startling in view of the frequency with which one hears that boys are favoured in that country. This surprising result is at least partly due to the fact that individual data are being measured against a standard that has a male advantage built into it. When the same data are measured against the presumably non-gender-biased NCHS standard, the apparent female advantage tends to disappear, although the expected male advantage still fails to become visible. We will return to the question of gender differences in nutrition in chapter 5. For present purposes, the important point is that the choice of reference population itself strongly affects the gender contrast we witness in anthropometry.

Relations among the hunger indicators

The assumption is sometimes made that patterns of variation or change observable in child anthropometry indicate variation or change in nutritional status for the population of all ages. The prevalence of underweight among small children is used as a leading indicator of malnutrition in famine early warning systems, and cross-sectional variations in underweight among small children are taken as indicators of likely concentrations of malnutrition at other ages as well. Little attempt seems to have been made to validate this wider application of the findings on child anthropometry by exploring its association with hunger indicators pertaining directly to other age groups. Given the crucial importance, for malnutrition among small children, of processes such as weaning and childhood diseases that are irrelevant to others, the use of childhood anthropometry as an indicator of nutritional conditions for adolescents and adults seems questionable.

As Heyer (1991) observed in her analysis of Kenyan data:

Child malnutrition is not at all closely linked with ... poverty (whether measured in terms of income or expenditure) ... or even food intake estimates. This is consistent with micro-level evidence on the role of health and other factors.

Similarly, for a low-income sample in the Philippines, Pinstrup-Andersen (1990) found only low correlations between child anthropometry and a wide range of household-level indicators – per capita household income, per capita food acquisition, per capita calorie consumption, household calorie adequacy, total household food acquisition, and total household calorie consumption. The highest correlation was only .22. The very weak relationships between child anthropometry and other hunger indicators suggest that children's growth impairment is not a useful indicator of household food security. The authors were actually asking the opposite question – whether household food-security indicators would serve to identify households in which malnourished children were located. The answer to this question was also negative. In contrast, caloric adequacy of pregnant and lactating women was reasonably strongly related to that of their households, suggesting that nutritional problems for this group are more a function of household food insecurity and also discounting the interpretation that poor measurement of household data could account for the lack of relationship with child anthropometry.

To identify linkages between individual and household hunger, which is essential for diagnosing nutrition problems and setting priorities for interventions, empirical work using data covering a broad range of ages and including multiple indicators of hunger needs to be given a high priority. Such work might explore, for example, the extent to which underweight children are concentrated in households with low access to food, and the covariation of anthropometry for children and adults within the same households. If it turns out that underweight among small children acts as a reliable proxy for hunger of others in the same household, location, or social group, the wide availability of childhood anthropometry could be exploited more systematically to enhance our overall understanding of hunger in entire populations. If, on the other hand, variations in childhood anthropometry diverge sharply from those reflected by other hunger indicators, the temptation to generalize widely from data pertaining directly only to small children should be resisted. In the meantime, it is safer to interpret *changes* in child anthropometry within a region or social class as indicative of changes in the hunger status of entire families, but not without first considering whether changes in infant feeding practices or in the disease environment might provide an adequate explanation for the trends.

Notes

1. The World Bank most commonly used a cut-off set at 90 per cent of the caloric requirements estimated by the FAO/WHO/UNU committee in 1971; the FAO defined its cut-off as 1.4 times the basal metabolic rate (BMR). In neither case do the cut-offs employed allow for more than minimal physical activity for adults, and the newer common cut-off of 1.54 BMR still allows only for light activity (Uvin 1994).
2. Counting breast-feeding bouts over shorter periods is problematic because daytime consumption may or may not be reflective of night-time consumption: when children sleep with their mothers, nursing may follow a similar pattern around the clock; where they do not, there may be little or no night-time nursing.
3. Sukhatme and Margen (1982) interpret interindividual variation observed cross-sectionally as reflecting intra-individual variability; they also interpret the autocorrelation of daily individual intakes as evidence of a homoeostatic, self-regulating process. Although neither of these interpretations is implausible, interindividual variation could reflect stable differences across individuals and autocorrelation of intakes could result from external influences that vary cyclically over a span of days (such as different eating patterns on weekends and weekdays). Even if the evidence for energy intake and efficiency of use as a self-regulating process were definitive, the conclusion that intake levels observed only as the low point in a fluctuating series could be maintained indefinitely without damage seems questionable.
4. Smallness on any of the anthropometric indicators may result from illness rather than from compromised nutrition, though in most cases it is likely to be a combination of the two. Smallness may also result from normal variation or genetic potential, and one of the challenges this presents is to set cut-off points for anthropometric measurements that identify nutritional problems without also including children who are simply small.
5. Mid-upper arm circumference has been shown to predict risk of death better than either weight for height or height for age (Briend et al. 1987).

Works cited

Ahn, Chung Hae, and William C. MacLean. 1980. "Growth of the Exclusively Breast-Fed Infant." *American Journal of Clinical Nutrition* 33: 183–192.

APS. 1992. *Nigeria's Census Confounds Experts*. All Africa Press Service, APS News Bulletin, 30 March. Nairobi, Kenya: All Africa Press Service.

Atwood, D. A. 1991. "Aggregate Food Supply and Famine Early Warning." *Food Policy* 16, No. 3: 245–251.

Beaton, G. H. 1989. "Small But Healthy? Are We Asking the Right Question?" *Human Organization* 48, No. 1: 30–38.

Briend, A., M. G. M. Rowland, and B. Wojtyniak. 1987. "Measures of Nutritional Status." *Lancet* 1, No. 8541: 1098–1099.

Cameron, M. E., and W. A. Van Staveren. 1988. *Manual on Methodology for Food Consumption Studies*. Oxford: Oxford University Press.

Chandra, R. K. 1982. "Physical Growth of Exclusively Breast-Fed Infants." *Nutrition Research* 2: 275–276.

Dasgupta, Partha, and Debraj Ray. 1990. "Adapting to Undernourishment: The Biological Evidence and its Implications." In: Jean Drèze and Amartya Sen, eds. *The Political Economy of Hunger*, Volume I. Oxford: Clarendon Press, pp. 191–246.

den Hartog, A. P. 1973. "Unequal Distribution of Food Within the Household (A Somewhat Neglected Aspect of Food Behaviour)." *FAO Nutrition Newsletter* 10, No. 4: 8–15.

Dibley, M. J., J. Goldsby, M. Strehling, and F. L. Trowbridge. 1987. "Development of Normalized Curves for the International Growth Reference: Historical and Technical Considerations." *American Journal of Clinical Nutrition* 46: 736–748.

FAO. 1977. *The Fourth World Food Survey*. Food and Nutrition Series. Rome: Food and Agriculture Organization of the United Nations.

———. 1983. *A Comparative Study of Food Consumption Data from Food Balance Sheets and Household Surveys*. FAO Economic and Social Development Paper No. 34. Rome: Food and Agriculture Organization of the United Nations.

———. 1984. *Food Balance Sheets 1979–81 Average*. Rome: Food and Agriculture Organization of the United Nations.

———. 1985. *The Fifth World Food Survey*. Food and Nutrition Series. Rome: Food and Agriculture Organization of the United Nations.

———. 1990a. "Action Programmes to Overcome Specific Nutritional Deficiencies in the Asia-Pacific Region." *Twentieth Regional Conference for Asia and the Pacific* in Beijing, China. Rome: Food and Agriculture Organization of the United Nations.

———. 1990b. "Malnutrition in the Latin American and Caribbean Region: Causes and Prevention." *Twenty-First Regional Conference for Latin America and the Caribbean* in Santiago, Chile. Rome: Food and Agriculture Organization of the United Nations.

———. 1990c. "Strategies for Combating Malnutrition in Africa." *Sixteenth FAO Regional Conference for Africa* in Accra, Ghana. Rome: Food and Agriculture Organization of the United Nations.

Garza, C., and N. F. Butte. 1990. "Energy Intakes of Human Milk-Fed Infants During the First Year." *Journal of Pediatrics* 117, No. 2: S124–S131.

Grant, James P. 1990. *The State of the World's Children 1990*. New York: Oxford University Press for UNICEF.

Heyer, J. 1991. "Poverty and Food Deprivation in Kenya's Smallholder Agricultural Areas." In: J. Drèze and A. Sen, eds. *The Political Economy of Hunger*, Volume III. Oxford: Clarendon Press.

Huffman, Sandra. 1991. "Maternal Malnutrition and Breastfeeding: Is There Really a Choice for Policy Makers?" *Journal of Tropical Pediatrics* 37, Suppl. 1: 19–22.

Jelliffe, Derrick B., and E. F. Patrice Jelliffe. 1989. *Community Nutritional Assessment: With Special Reference to Less Technically Developed Countries*. Oxford Medical Publications. Oxford: Oxford University Press.

Katona-Apte, Judit. 1975. "The Relevance of Nourishment to the Reproductive Cycle of the Female in India." In: Dana Raphael, ed. *Being Female: Reproduction, Power, and Change*. The Hague: Mouton, pp. 43–48.

Laderman, Carol. 1991. "Where the Wild Things Are." In: Anne Sharman, Janet Theophano, Karen Curtis, and Ellen Messer, eds. *Diet and Domestic Life in Society.* Philadelphia: Temple University Press, pp. 15–32.

Maher, Vanessa. 1981. "Work, Consumption and Authority with the Household." In: Kate Young, Carol Wolkowitz, and Roslyn McCullagh, eds. *Of Marriage and the Market: Women's Subordination in International Perspective.* London: CSE Books, pp. 69–87.

Martorell, Reynaldo. 1995. "Promoting Healthy Growth: Rationale and Benefits." In: Per Pinstrup-Andersen, David Pelletier, and Harold Alderman, eds. *Child Growth and Nutrition in Developing Countries.* Ithaca: Cornell University Press, pp. 15–31.

Messer, Ellen. 1986. "The 'Small But Healthy' Hypothesis: Historical, Political, and Ecological Influences on Nutritional Standards." *Human Ecology* 14, No. 1: 57–75.

Millman, Sara Ruth, and Robert S. Chen. 1991. *Measurement of Hunger: Defining Thresholds.* RR-91-1. Providence, Rhode Island: Alan Shawn Feinstein World Hunger Program.

———, ———, J. Emlen, V. Haarmann, Jeanne X. Kasperson, and Ellen Messer. 1991. *The Hunger Report: Update 1991.* HR-91-1. Providence, Rhode Island: Alan Shawn Feinstein World Hunger Program.

Mosley, W. Henry, and Lincoln C. Chen. 1984. "An Analytic Framework for the Study of Child Survival in Developing Countries." *Population and Development Review* 10 (Suppl.): 25–48.

National Research Council. 1986. *Nutrient Adequacy: Assessment Using Food Consumption Surveys.* Washington, D.C.: National Academy Press.

NNMB. 1981. *Report for the Year 1980.* Hyderabad, India: National Institute of Nutrition.

———. 1989. *Interim Report of Repeat Survey (Phase I) 1988–89.* Hyderabad, India: National Institute of Nutrition.

Osmani, S. R. 1992. "On Some Controversies in the Measurement of Under-nutrition." In: S. R. Osmani, ed. *Nutrition and Poverty.* Oxford: Clarendon Press, pp. 121–164.

Papanek, Hanna. 1990. "To Each Less Than She Needs, From Each More Than She Can Do: Allocations, Entitlements, and Value." In: Irene Tinker, ed. *Persistent Inequalities: Women in World Development.* New York: Oxford University Press, pp. 162–181.

Pinstrup-Andersen, P. 1990. "Data on Food Consumption by High-Risk Family Members: Its Utility for Identifying Target Households for Food and Nutrition Programmes." In: B. L. Rogers and N. P. Schlossman, eds. *Intra-Household Resource Allocation: Issues and Methods for Development Policy and Planning.* Tokyo: United Nations University Press, pp. 164–175.

Popkin, Barry M. 1994. "The Nutrition Transition in Low Income Countries: An Emerging Crisis." *Nutrition Reviews* 52, No. 9: 285–298.

Puffer, R. R., and C. V. Serrano. 1973. *Patterns of Mortality in Childhood.* Pan American Health Organization, Scientific Publication No. 262. Washington, D.C.: PAHO.

Ritchie, C. D., and D. J. Naismith. 1975. "A Comparison of Growth in Wholly Breast-Fed Infants and in Artificially Fed Infants." *Proceedings of the Nutrition Society* 34, No. 3: 118A.

Scrimshaw, N. S., and V. R. Young. 1989. "Adaptation to Low Protein and Energy Intakes." *Human Organization* 48, No. 1: 20–29.

Stuff, Janice E., and Buford L. Nichols. 1989. "Nutrient Intake and Growth Performance of Older Infants Fed Human Milk." *Journal of Pediatrics* 115: 959–968.

Sukhatme, P. V. 1988. "Energy Intake and Nutrition: On the Autoregulatory Homeostatic Nature of Energy Balance." In: T. N. Srinivasan and Pranab K. Bardhan, eds. *Rural Poverty in South Asia.* New York: Columbia University Press, pp. 365–388.

Svedberg, P. 1991. "Undernutrition in Sub-Saharan Africa: A Critical Assessment of the Evidence." In: J. Drèze and A. K. Sen, eds. *The Political Economy of Hunger.* Volume III. Oxford: Oxford University Press.

THP. 1983. "Where We Stand Today" (Editorial). *The Hunger Project* 17: 6–7.

Tomkins, A., and F. Watson. 1989. *Malnutrition and Infection: A Review.* United Nations, Administrative Committee on Coordination, Subcommittee on Nutrition, ACC/SCN State-of-the-Art Series Discussion Paper No. 5. Geneva: World Health Organization.

Underwood, B. A., and Y. Hofvander. 1982. "Appropriate Timing for Complementary Feeding of the Breast-fed Infant: A Review." *Acta Paediatrica Scandinavica* Suppl. 294.

UNDP. 1992. *Human Development Report 1992.* United Nations Development Programme. New York: Oxford University Press.

Uvin, Peter. 1994. "The State of World Hunger." *Nutrition Reviews* 52, No. 5: 151–161.

Waterlow, J. C. 1989. "Observations on the FAP's Methodology for Estimating the Incidence of Undernutrition." *Food and Nutrition Bulletin* 11, No. 2: 8–13.

Whitehead, R. G., and A. A. Paul. 1984. "Growth Charts and the Assessment of Infant Feeding Practices in the Western World and in Developing Countries." *Early Human Development* 9: 187–207.

WHO. 1985. *Energy and Protein Requirements. Report of a Joint FAO/WHO/UNU Expert Consultation.* World Health Organization, Technical Report Series 724. Geneva: WHO.

Wilson, Christine S. 1974. "Child Following: A Technique for Learning Food and Nutrient Intakes." *Journal of Tropical Pediatrics and Environmental Child Health* 20: 9–14.

World Bank. 1992. *World Development Report 1992: Development and the Environment.* New York: Oxford University Press for the World Bank.

3

Food shortage

Ellen Messer and Laurie F. DeRose

Food shortage occurs when food supplies within a bounded region do not provide the energy and nutrients needed by that region's population. Food shortage is most easily conceptualized as a production problem – not enough food is grown to meet regional needs – but constraints on importation as well as storage can also cause or contribute to food shortage. Food shortage is also created where food is exported from areas where production is adequate or even abundant. Historically, the great hunger of Ireland (1845–1847) and the famine of Bengal (1944) have been attributed more to British political decisions to export locally produced grain supplies without compensating imports than to production shortfalls *per se* (Woodham-Smith 1962; Sen 1981).

Even when production shortfall is the primary cause of insufficient supply, the ecological and political reasons for production problems vary widely. They range from natural disasters such as drought, flood, or fungus, to political disasters such as civil conflict, to misguided economic policies such as price controls – all of which discourage production of essential foods.

In all situations of food shortage, many within the region's population are hungry; but in every food-short region, others still enjoy adequate access to food. Equally, although many are food secure in areas of adequate food production, some still go hungry. These variable patterns of hunger result not only from skewed food distribution within regions based on differential political and economic resources, but also from selective marketing, and from non-market political policies of food extraction or assistance.

This chapter begins with an overview of the evidence for global and regional food shortage and where it is most likely to occur. It then analyses the causes of country or within-country food shortages. Finally, it considers the relationship between drought and famine, using recent evidence to argue that food shortage is not inevitable even in areas of widespread production failures: political, not environmental factors are the primary causes of food shortages. This message is repeated in chapter 6, which addresses food shortage caused by armed conflict.

Is there a world food shortage?

World agriculture produces enough food calories to meet the energy needs of all the nearly 6 billion (6×10^9) people who are alive today. Increased production based on advances in seed, water, and environmental technologies, and their wider dissemination especially in developing countries, have removed insufficient production as a cause of food shortage for the world as a whole. Global agriculture has managed to keep pace with population growth, and world food security is also safeguarded by cereal carry-over stocks; 19–20 per cent of annual cereal consumption is carried over into the next year to provide food in case of disastrous production failure (FAO 1993).[1] Nevertheless, during any year in which enough calories are produced on a global level to meet the energy requirements of the entire population, food shortages can still occur under two situations. If the patterning of production directs too many calories into animals instead of humans, some enjoy meat while others lack calories. Alternatively, overemphasis on production of calories may jeopardize the production of other protein- or micronutrient-rich foods that also enter into the calculus of global food security or shortage. Both are production as well as distribution issues.

Dietary factors in world food shortage

The numbers of people potentially supported by the global food supply depend heavily on the kind of diet people consume. The World Hunger Program calculates that global food supplies have been more than adequate, since the mid-1970s, to support the world's population on a vegetarian diet (table 3.1). But they would support only 74 per cent of the 1993 population on a diet where 15 per cent of calories come from animal foods (Uvin 1996). Only 56 per cent of the 1993

Table 3.1 **Numbers of people supported by 1993 global food supply with different diets**

Diet	Population potentially supported by 1993 food supply	
	Billion	Percentage of world population
Near-vegetarian	6.26	112
With 15% of calories from animal foods	4.12	74
With 25% of calories from animal foods	3.16	56

Source: adapted from Uvin (1996)

world population could have been provided with diets where 25 per cent of calories came from animal foods (Uvin 1996).

Vegetarian diets are typical in a wide range of developing countries, but worldwide the demand for meat is growing. Diets in industrialized countries differ widely with respect to their composition: those living in the United Kingdom eat less meat per capita than residents of the United States; meat consumption in Sweden is only 60 per cent of the US average (Bender 1994). Beef production continues to increase and poultry production is increasing faster than population growth rates. Although the *rate* of growth in the production of animal foods has been slower since 1980 than in the previous few decades, production of these foods continues to increase (Wisner and Wang 1990). Food shortage of the future, calculated on the basis of total future demand for grain consumed directly or in the form of animal foods, will be conditioned by whether peoples adopting richer diets follow the European or US pathway.

Food security must also take into account the growing demand for higher-cost cereals such as rice and wheat over sorghum and root-crops, as well as animal products. All are more resource expensive to produce. Increased demand for meat is a particular concern, since livestock conversions, usually calculated in terms of food energy grain-to-livestock ratios, are high. In a feedlot, it takes two kilos (kilograms) of grain to produce one kilo of chicken or fish, four kilos to produce one kilo of pork, and seven to produce one kilo of beef. Some suggest the ratios may be even higher: 3:1, 6:1, and 16:1. In the 1990s, it was calculated that some 4.3 billion large domesticated animals and 17 billion poultry eat 40 per cent of the world's grain supply (Foster 1992). Animal production also takes land and water resources. The argument can be made that these might be allocated otherwise to less resource-expensive food crops, but the livestock economy is complex, and reductions in animal production will not produce more food suddenly at lower cost.

Food shortage also coincides with adequate calorie production where the foods consumed are deficient in protein or micronutrients. Diets may be adequate in quantity but not quality. The three most common micronutrient deficiencies, those of iron, iodine, and vitamin A, are described in the Introduction to this volume (chapter 1). Such deficiencies are most common in vegetarian or near-vegetarian diets that lack variety, both because such diets tend to be consumed by people who lack resources to acquire greater variety and because some nutrients are more abundant in animal foods.

Strategies to change consumption patterns

These failures of the global food system to prevent food shortage despite adequate food energy production are being addressed in various ways in both developed and developing countries. In developed countries, higher consumption of animal foods is being discouraged. Meat consumption has begun to decline in response to health concerns that diets high in animal fat contribute to cardiovascular disease and certain cancers. Nutritionists are also trying to improve the dietary habits of poorer people, who tend to consume diets higher in fat. For reasons of equity and conservation, "food first," ecology, and natural resource advocates in developed countries also stress the importance of "eating low on the food chain" – more grain and vegetables, less meat – to make more food available to meet global food needs, and to encourage sustainable agricultural practices (Lappe 1991; Brown and Kane 1994).

To meet world food needs, fat consumption also needs to be discouraged in some developing countries where average meat consumption is still at relatively healthy levels, but demands for animal protein and fats are increasing.[2] Increasing the consumption of grains, legumes, root crops, and vegetables, relative to animal products, involves changing dietary patterns in developed countries and reversing current trends toward higher consumption of meat and fats in developing countries. Since higher status conventionally is associated with greater meat and fat consumption, such dietary change challenges traditional social, as well as nutritional, beliefs and practices and may prove difficult.

Micronutrient deficiencies, by contrast, can be targeted by a number of specific interventions: (1) increasing intake of foods containing them; (2) fortifying or enriching other foods so that they contain more of the needed nutrients, or (3) providing oral or injectable vitamins and minerals. To be successful, however, all rely on some degree of political commitment, as well as behavioural change. Although costs for some programmes are relatively low (e.g. salt iodization costs only about five cents per person per year, and vitamin A capsules only about six cents [Grant 1995]), they demand technical and social organization, and political and community support, for effective implementation and monitoring.

Despite these concerns about dietary quality, the most important conclusion to be drawn from an analysis of global food shortage is that there is no such shortage. Hunger is not primarily caused by food shortage.

Where are there regional food shortages?

Although global food production has kept pace with world population growth, the rate of population growth has outstripped the rate of growth in food production significantly in some developing regions, and caused per capita food availability in these regions to decline. Per capita food production in developing countries overall has increased less than 10 per cent since 1960, despite impressive continued growth in *total* food production. Trends in food production are the worst in sub-Saharan Africa (SSA), where per capita food production has decreased slowly but relentlessly in recent years. Developed countries over this same period were able to increase both food production and production per capita, however, benefiting from advancing technology but also much lower population growth rates than in developing countries.

Per capita food availability has remained relatively constant in food-deficit regions and countries, primarily owing to food imports acquired through trade or aid (ACC/SCN 1993). FAO estimates of dietary energy supply (DES), which not only measure net food production (minus exports) and imports but also account for food lost, stored, or used for animal feed or industry, show that in only two regions – SSA and South Asia – does DES per capita fall below basic average requirements (set at 2250 calories [table 3.2]). High fertility combined with underdeveloped agricultural technology and infrastructure, plus high incidence of natural disasters and civil disorder,

Table 3.2 **Per capita dietary energy supply by region, 1990**

Region	Calories	Region	Calories
Sub-Saharan Africa	2,099	Near East and North Africa	3,094
South Asia	2,245	Oceania	3,330
South-East Asia	2,446	Former USSR	3,380
South America	2,625	Europe	3,450
China	2,657	North America	3,600
Central America	2,822		

Source: Uvin (1994), compiled from ACC/SCN (1993: 119) and FAO (1992: 21).

make SSA the region most evidently food short. In South Asia, even though birth rates and population growth have slowed and agricultural output has increased dramatically in South Asia over the past two decades, there is still not enough food to ensure adequate nourishment for everyone.

Two lessons that can be drawn from these low-DES regions are that severe production shortfalls are not so easily made up by food imports, and that population growth is not the only cause of food shortage.

In SSA, low DES is often attributed to low import capacity due to low export earnings and large burden of debt service. But even were these constraints removed, there would remain those of low economic (including agricultural) productivity, civil strife, and lack of infrastructure. Greater dependence on imports within the region would also magnify associated logistical problems – higher costs per unit food as demand increases, transportation costs to reach remoter areas, expanded costs of shipping, and storage losses. Multiplying numbers of conflicts and their aftermaths already have created unmet demand for food aid, especially as the costs of the actual food increase in an environment of shrinking foreign assistance.

In South Asia, the data indicate that food shortage remains a key issue, even where per capita food production has continued to rise along with population increase. Per capita DES has increased steadily in South Asia since 1970, despite very modest gains in per capita income (Uvin 1994). Even if lower caloric requirements are accepted for South Asians, based on their smaller body size (see controversy described in chapter 2), there are further signs of food shortage in this region.

Additional indicators of food shortage in both of these regions are provided by the World Food Programme, which has carried out far more emergency operations in SSA than elsewhere; their next most heavily aided region is Asia (Uvin 1994). Emergencies refer to both man-made and natural disasters. Furthermore, in these two regions, *each* of the three major micronutrient deficiency diseases is a serious public health problem, as contrasted with other regions that suffer from one or two but not all. Their combined food and nutritional deficiencies contribute to a continuing cycle of low productivity and hunger in the countries of these regions.

How common are country-level food shortages?

Global and even regional food availability estimates hide important variations in DES and food self-sufficiency of individual countries. Although Latin America as a whole has more than enough food to feed the region's population, seven countries in the region (with populations totalling 67.2 million people) had DES below requirement over the period from 1988 to 1990 (UNDP 1994). There are an additional 13.6 million people living in countries with inadequate food availability, despite being in regions where food supply is adequate. The remaining 721.5 million people living in hungry countries also live in hungry regions (Uvin 1996).

Food self-sufficiency is an additional issue and a potential determinant of food shortage. "Food First" advocates have argued that the only way for a country to prevent hunger is to promote food self-sufficiency or self-reliance (countries are able to trade for quantities sufficient to meet home country needs [Lappe and Collins 1978]). In their analysis, the country that lacks food self-sufficiency is a hungry country or, in our current terms, food short. Fortunately, the data do not support this oversimplification. Of the 99 countries that did not produce enough food to meet the needs of their national populations in the 1980s, only 48 (32 in SSA) were food short as measured by per capita DES (Uvin 1994). Thus, a country's dependence on imported food does not necessarily mean that more people in the country are hungry or that the country has exhausted its agricultural potential. Small industrial food-importing countries easily produce enough other goods to cover the costs of their food needs, purchased on the world market.

However, Lappe and Collins's assessment may be correct for countries with predominantly poor rural agricultural economies. The failure of a city-state such as Hong Kong to grow enough to feed its urban population has hunger implications that differ greatly from the failures of predominantly rural African countries whose export earnings are low. For poor agricultural populations, whose entitlements to food may come in large part from home production, their country's deteriorating position of food self-sufficiency may be an indicator of their own reduced access to food and resources to produce food.

Causes of shortage

The discussion above on prevalence and indicators of food shortage has illustrated that its causes are complex. Some hunger indicators, such as production shortfalls, highlight problems that *may* lead to food shortage. Others, such as DES, directly measure food availability within a country or region. These food-shortage indicators report outcomes of physical and biological factors, sociocultural influences, political-economic forces, and interactions among these elements.

Physical and biological factors

Production is only one determinant of food shortage, but a crucial one. It is obviously critical on the global level but can also be decisive for some countries or communities. Production potential varies across countries, dependent on natural factors (including climate, soils, water, food species, and pests) and cultural factors (including technology and investment strategies).

Climate
Temperature and rainfall are critical elements determining when and how often crops can be sown. While some Asian countries are able to harvest three times in a single year, food production nearly halts during dry seasons in many tropical zones and during winter cold in temperate areas. Extremes or thresholds of heat, increasingly accompanied by high ultraviolet radiation, and of cold, especially early frosts or late thaws, can ruin harvests. They test the limits of growing seasons and moisture–temperature tolerances of particular crop varieties. These extremes will be modified by global climate change, which promises to transform regional cropping patterns. For the present, drought is the most widespread climatic threat to production, and is treated more extensively below.

Seasonality means that there may be food shortage during part of the year in places where total annual production appears to be more than sufficient to meet nutritional needs. Agricultural societies and households adapt to potential seasonal scarcities by planting a variety of early- to later-yielding crops, storing or selling harvests to minimize losses, investing in social feasting when food is plentiful, and drawing on social obligations of reciprocity when food is scarce. They ration, process food staples more coarsely, supplement diets through foraging, and consume less-preferred foods. They also schedule crafts, migrant labour, and other economic activities to diversify and ensure income in "off" agricultural seasons. Despite such adaptive mechanisms, prolonged or multiple years of shortage, as experienced especially in SSA and South Asia, give rise to potential famine conditions (defined as widespread and extreme food shortage leading to elevated mortality and mass movements of population in search of food) that nowadays are addressed relatively successfully by state and international early warning systems (EWS) and response. Even where EWS are well established (as in India), however, seasonal hunger remains a problem addressed neither by state nor by traditional sociocultural mechanisms of food sharing, which tend to be undermined by modernization (Chen 1991).

Although drought is often thought of as the precipitating cause of famine, because so many farmers in a single area experience crop failure simultaneously, drought does not lead to food shortage or its extreme manifestation – famine – if there are adequate carry-over stocks available, or if food is available through market or relief channels (Ravallion 1987).

Creeping disasters, such as drought, are likely to devastate crops but leave infrastructure intact. Both timing and duration of rainfall may be implicated, since, for seed crops, moisture is critical immediately after planting and also at the stages when fertilizer is applied. Drought can also prevent planting if the rains are late, so that soils are too dry to till before the planting season has passed. Failure of rains at any of these stages greatly reduces harvests.

Since the early origins of agriculture, human societies have always tried to extend productive seasons and, especially, available moisture by controlling groundwater evapotranspiration, by various water-storage techniques, and by distribution via irrigation. Water control is closely linked to social power and control, since the ability of irrigation systems to enhance food production is limited by their general state of repair. Hydraulic systems, which initially require large amounts of capital and labour to construct, later require maintenance. Social resources must be mobilized through a sense of common purpose (or coercion) to preserve irrigation ways, which other-

61

wise silt up, leak, and lose effectiveness. The history of political fortunes and social breakdown in the Near East and Middle East has been linked to cycles of "salt and silt," environmental and subsistence crises triggered by failures to control the life-giving waters of irrigation (Jacobsen and Adams 1955). The expansion and sustainability of Green Revolution (GR) agriculture in the modern era is similarly dependent on effective water management, which is necessary to prevent waterlogging and salinization of soils and crops, and silting and disruption of water channels.

At the opposite end of the rainfall spectrum, too much rain can also impair agricultural production, especially where flooding is severe enough to kill crops by uprooting or submergence, but also where it simply slows growths or makes cultivation and harvesting extremely difficult. Even after harvest, flooding can be devastating when it occurs before crops have been safely stored (Good 1986) and leaves crops vulnerable to rot.

Irrigation systems can be overloaded by flooding but also can be one of the mechanisms used to cope with irregular rainfall. Irrigation systems often do little to prevent damage caused by the force of the rains themselves but they do prevent further damage from waterlogging. They also enhance productivity in dry seasons by holding over water from heavy rains; this is accomplished through the use of simple earthen dams in Sri Lanka (Grigg 1985), as well as through more elaborate systems of canals and pumps. Along with terracing, irrigation systems may also limit soil erosion and help sustain soil fertility along flood plains.

Less regularly, food systems can be entirely disrupted by natural disasters, which affect both growing and marketing conditions and sometimes the social fabric. Hurricanes and, to a lesser extent, earthquakes can destroy crops. They can also devastate transport, markets, and other infrastructure, and cause food shortage even where the crops themselves survive. The economic destruction accompanying natural disasters, which can cause scarcities of many materials, often pushes prices upward, increasing the rate of inflation, reducing employment, and more generally contributing to balance-of-payments problems.

Inability of government to deal effectively with natural disaster, such as earthquake or drought, can threaten political stability and overturn fragile regimes. In each of the recent cases of Ethiopia, the Sudan, and Rwanda, their ruling governments' ineffectiveness in dealing with drought and ensuing famine conditions provided an opening for the political opposition to challenge successfully that government's authority and legitimacy. Political leaders were portrayed as prospering while the masses went hungry, and this became the successful rallying point for civil uprisings. Similarly, the inability of Samoza's regime in Nicaragua to alleviate widespread suffering from a hurricane became the trigger cause of the Sandanista's successful ascent to political power. Each case, however, was followed by periods of readjustment, civil disorder, and lowered food productivity.

Although the magnitude of disasters' effects on overall economic development appears to vary (Albala-Bertrand 1993), the short-term economic shocks caused by sudden natural disasters usually decrease marketed food availability in the affected regions, so that food aid may appear to be the only practical means of getting enough food to the affected populations. Inappropriate world response, such as Guatemala's inundation with donated food following the 1976 earthquake, sometimes disrupts markets and income for local farmers, who face plummeting food prices and agricultural income even where their crops have not been destroyed. The question of whether food aid increases food availability at the household level will be revisited in chapter 4.

Politicians and national politics are also important social actors in other ways. They provide the economic, social, and cultural framework (what policy makers increasingly term "the enabling environment") to prevent natural elements from precipitating wider disasters. Despite the seemingly arbitrary nature of sudden natural disasters, they do not affect all areas in the same way, even when their severity is of a similar scale. Healthy economies rapidly bounce back from shocks because they have more internal resources dedicated to mitigating the immediate and longer-term impacts on food production or distribution. Similarly, precautions that minimize the impact of disasters, such as earthquake-resistant housing and roads, are not distributed evenly either across or within countries. Some so-called "natural" disasters might be better thought of as man made. For example, flooding often results as much from deforestation as from excessive rainfall or unusually intense hurricanes. Abuse of land, particularly overgrazing, increases vulnerability to wind and flood erosion (Albala-Bertrand 1993). Sudden natural disasters cannot be prevented, but the effects that they have on food production and food importation are conditioned more by political and economic processes than by the intensity of the calamity.

Soils

Food production also varies according to soil structure and fertility, factors that are less easily measured – but perhaps more easily modified – than temperature or rainfall. The differences in productivity between the dark soils of the US midwest and the sands of the Sahara appear obvious, but it is less clear how much less-dramatic variations in soil conditions matter. Many tropical soils contain less nitrogen and phosphorus, have lower capacity to absorb fertilizers, and therefore have lower conventional productive capacity, but some tropical soils (most notably in the Amazon) have been very intensively farmed and further intensification is possible in other areas (NAS 1986).

Since agricultural methods and inputs vary in areas with different soils, the causes of disparities in productivity are multiple. Grain yields per hectare in SSA are about one-third of those achieved in East Asia, but SSA also struggles with more challenging climate, uses fertilizer at a rate less than 13 per cent of the world average (World Bank 1992), and has made little use of irrigation. Investments in agricultural intensification, including higher-yield-potential seeds, fertilizers, water management, and chemicals for pest control, are costly and make it unlikely that they will be easily or widely available for use by poorer farmers and countries. Especially where imported food is cheaper than domestically produced food, as is the case today in many developing countries, expanding local production may not appear to be economically feasible.

Production may also be limited by low soil fertility and restricted access to fertilizer supplies. Fertilizer is required to realize the full benefits from hybrid GR seeds; quantities of its use often serve as a measure of agricultural improvement or modernization. In contrast to the time when most farmers used local sources of animal or green manure to enhance soil fertility, most developing countries today rely heavily on inorganic fertilizers, which they must import. At both household and country levels, fertilizer constitutes a significant expense, and lack of means to purchase adequate quantities potentially reduces crop yields. Lack of cash, poor credit, or isolation from sources of supply due to underdeveloped infrastructure hamper farmers' access; lack of foreign exchange and balance-of-payments difficulties limit the total supplies imported and available within a country. The cost per unit of fertilizer is also a factor adding to the gap between fertilizer needs and the amount that many developing countries can afford to import (Monteón 1982; UNCTAD and

Mukherjee 1985). Upward fluctuations in the price of petroleum, a raw material for inorganic fertilizers, imperilled developing country food production in the mid-1970s, and could happen again. Timely, as well as total, availability constrains output, since optimal fertilizer impact is achieved only by applying it at the most sensitive points in the crop cycle. Only greater domestic production can protect farmers and consumers in developing countries from severe price fluctuations and transport or market bottlenecks.

Biological stressors
Disease, insects, animals, and weeds also damage crops and reduce yields, and are controlled by mechanical, land management, chemical, or biological means, including breeding plants and animals to resist key stressors.

Viruses are controlled by eliminating insect or other vectors and by breeding resistant seeds through conventional or new genetic engineering techniques. Biotechnology also offers new diagnostic techniques for identifying and limiting infections, as well as for producing and multiplying clean seeding stocks for vegetatively propagated crops, such as potatoes and manioc. Diagnostics and planting-material multiplication potentially can be carried out as local-level cottage industries. Bacterial and fungal diseases are also addressed through breeding programmes and sometimes chemical applications. In addition to the breeding and selection of resistant stock, animal diseases are controlled by preventive inoculations and curative remedies. Biological and chemical control of vectors are also common, and sometimes innovative, as where scientists of the Kenya-based International Centre of Insect Physiology and Ecology developed a simple cow urine-baited trap for tsetse flies, to eliminate trypanosomes.

Insect damage similarly is avoided by breeding resistant varieties, mixed-planting strategies that buffer particular host species from their characteristic pests, and insecticidal chemicals that kill (or otherwise interfere with the feeding, maturation, or sexual reproduction of) the target populations. Biological controls involve introducing predators or pathogens of the pest species. Integrated pest management that combines chemical, biological, and some hands-on mechanical strategies – such as removal of insect eggs before they hatch – are increasing worldwide, in response in part to their greater safety and lower costs and in part to the increasing environmental burden and decreasing effectiveness of chemicals. Chemical use soared during the early decades of the GR, as new seeds were accompanied by chemical

65

packages that sometimes indiscriminately wiped out "good" as well as "bad" insects, removing the predators as well as pests, presenting an unprecedented opportunity for pesticide-resistant insects that co-evolved with the plants and chemicals in these GR ecosystems to cause severe crop damage. To restore insect ecology, reduce pesticide poisoning, and re-create a safer balance for plants and humans, Indonesia, as a case in point, banned most pesticides. On Java, in some seasons and places where rice-hopper damage can be anticipated to be enormous, communities have organized massive brigades of farmers and schoolchildren to collect the insects' eggs and so prevent damage (Indonesian National IPM Program 1991).

Other kinds of animal damage, such as that of rodents, birds, or livestock, are conventionally limited by human labour, although the "excess" child labour that traditionally scared birds and livestock from ripening fields is disappearing as schooling competes with agricultural tasks. Reduced child-labour availability is one of the factors leading to the selection of maize over sorghum in many parts of Africa, since maize ears are covered and less subject to damage than sorghum seeds, which are exposed. Rodent pests may be chased, physically killed, or poisoned, although the poisons are still not well controlled. Human poisoning is a hazard in cases of insecticides and rodent poisons, since the toxic chemicals tend to be sold in small quantities and not handled with the care specified by their manufacturers. The usual way to prevent larger animals stealing crops is scrupulous tending in areas where such risks are high.

Weed damage also is increasing, as plagues such as *Striga* spread across the maize and sorghum fields of Africa. Weeds choke out useful plants and also compete with cultivated plantings for soil nutrients and water, reducing their yields and disease/insect resistance. Careful plantings, to give the intended food crop a healthy start, or herbicides are alternative strategies, as less labour is available to hand-weed at very low wages. Seeds of major crops that have been genetically engineered to resist a particular brand of herbicide also are being aggressively developed and marketed by large chemical giants, such as Monsanto, that have purchased seed companies and the molecular-biologist/plant-breeding scientists to advance the match and ensure a continuing market for their chemicals. These developments, although they may increase crop production, also increase the chemical load and the potential for herbicide-resistant genes (traits) to pass from the desirable species to closely related weed species, which would then be equipped to inflict even more damage.

Two modern agricultural factors contributing to greater risk of pest damage are genetic uniformity and uniform or continuous cropping cycles. As most farmers in a region purchase the same single varieties of improved seeds designed to maximize production on the same agricultural cycles, they establish conditions ideal for the explosion of many pests. An overall strategy to reduce plant damage therefore is diversified cropping. Carefully patterned plantings of multiple species and varieties within species is a good hedge and an aspect of traditional agricultural practices that modern cultivators need to review.

Seeds and related technologies
Basic to all production strategies and yields are the seeds, which may be more or less productive; drought and disease resistant; or responsive to moisture, fertilizer, and other chemical inputs. In many regions, "traditional" seed varieties are less and less plentiful because they are unable to keep up with demand for more food and more intensive methods. Modern seeds, bred for shorter growing periods and neutral photoperiod, allow multiple sowings and harvests; they also may be tailored to resist insects and plagues that attack traditional varieties and lower their yields.

Exponential growth in world food production over the past three decades has been made possible largely by new seeds and related technological advances that have greatly increased output per unit of land and labour. The impact of the GR seed–water–chemical technologies on grain yields has greatly reduced food shortage, especially in rice- and wheat-growing regions. But technological advance can prevent food shortage only if (1) it continues to increase yields faster than the population grows, (2) food availability within agriculturally modernizing regions actually increases, and (3) increased caloric availability is not transformed into richer diets.

Controversy rages over whether the dramatic food production increases achieved over 1960–1990 are sustainable and will be able to keep up with projected population growth. Brown and Kane (1994), who think that world population has reached its agricultural limits, argue that prior to the GR there existed a backlog of agricultural technologies waiting to be applied. Today, by contrast, no such "breakthrough" technologies are waiting "on the shelf"; although advancing biotechnologies promise to enhance production, they will not allow the quantum jumps in production necessary to keep pace with growing population. Technological optimists, such as World Bank economists Mitchell and Ingco (1993), differ: they argue that biotechnologies hold very great potential to increase food supplies and that careful pricing of both factors of production and resulting food products also can stimulate more food production. Intermediate positions, such as that of the International Food Policy Research Institute (IFPRI) "2020 Vision for Food, Agriculture, and Environment," argue that there also exists greater potential than Brown and Kane allow, to expand the applications of known technologies to prevent regional shortages, but that the world community must make such agricultural investments their priority. Because of required investments and economies of scale, many poorer farmers in developing countries have not been able to take full advantage of existing technologies. Increasing food production in some areas may depend more on altering social and institutional structures to allow fuller utilization of existing technology; it depends less on radical new breakthroughs.

Other intermediate positions suggest that there exists great potential for significant reductions in expenditures, and increases in available food supplies, by controlling waste all through the food system (Bender 1994). Post-harvest losses in cereals are coming under control (Good 1986; Donahaye and Messer 1992) but those of roots, tubers, fruits, and vegetables remain very high: losses of potatoes are estimated at 5–40 per cent and of bananas at 20–80 per cent (Toma et al. 1991). Biotechnology can also contribute to reductions in loss over the entire cultivation cycle and after harvest (Donahaye and Messer 1992).

Such savings and incremental production will not automatically eliminate food shortage for hungry populations, however. Technological advances still need to be directed toward crops and cropping characteristics, and distributed in manners that benefit those vulnerable to hunger. A case in point is Mexico, which has continued to suffer food shortage despite more than doubling its food production over 1960–1985, a period over which the volume of imported grain increased more than 20-fold (Barkin et al. 1990). This massive increase in imports, concurrent with rapid expansion of domestic production, can be accounted for in part by the shift of land out of maize production and into sorghum. Although sorghum is a basic food crop consumed in many areas of the world, in Mexico it is used primarily for animal food and therefore actually contributed to domestic food shortage because of the associated drop in maize production and export of livestock.

In sum, food production, supply, and the productive environment are influenced by a range of physical and biological factors that are not easily separable from sociocultural and political-economic conditions. These illustrate the linkages between production and consumption at local, country, and global levels.

Social and cultural factors

The causes of food shortage are in no way limited to physical and biological factors affecting production. Sociocultural factors include the organization of land and labour use as well as dietary preferences. Political-economic factors involve world markets and government policies to modernize agriculture and increase foreign exchange, which at the local level are translated into incentive structures, especially "getting the prices right." Armed conflict, a major contributor to food shortage, is treated more extensively in chapter 6.

Land and water control

Land tenure greatly influences what and how much is grown. Motivations to invest in land improvements and agricultural technology are tied to anticipated returns from land ownership or rents. Land reform is often cited as the major policy tool to improve food and other agricultural output, but may be most difficult to implement, since it threatens vested interests. Barraclaugh (1989), in his probing analysis of policies to end hunger, found that even allegedly reformist governments, such as the Sandinistas in Nicaragua, are stymied by vested landholding power interests if they seek more equitable land allocations. Communal or private ownership, permanent or usufruct use rights, and tax or labour obligations associated with tenure are three kinds of conditions that define the social and political order and the social relations of production and consumption. Inequality in landholding is an index of social inequality: aggregate landholding (small to large) is used as a measure of household poverty or wealth and a predictor of household agricultural and economic productivity, food self-sufficiency, food insecurity, and technology adoption. Intolerably severe or growing inequality in landholding, experienced by peasant cultivators as denial of basic subsistence rights, has been the cause of most peasant revolutions of the twentieth century (Wolf 1969). Their struggle for land encompasses the larger struggle for individual and communal human dignity, political autonomy and identity, and a decent standard of living. The political violence and discrimination that precede conflict, the destructiveness of active conflict, and the difficulty of restoring communities and reconstructing food systems following conflict, are probably the most significant causes of food shortage and related poverty and deprivation. They are dealt with further below and in chapter 6.

The most important way in which landholding affects food supply is in the choice of crops. Plantation or latifundia systems in Central America historically have focused on cash crops for export, with smallholdings for food to meet subsistence needs. Indigenous cultivators in Guatemala historically were pushed off the most productive lands into mountainous refuge zones; in El Salvador, subsistence holdings were reduced to allow larger holdings for coffee. Struggle for land by former combatants as well as non-combatants in the former war zones of Guatemala, El Salvador, and Nicaragua remains a threat to political stability and future food self-reliance, as indigenous and peasant communities try to regroup, establish rights over land, and produce a mix of subsistence and cash crops for internal and external markets. On the island of Negros in the Philippines, large landholders employed peons to farm sugar. Landlords did not allow workers to convert land-use to subsistence production, even after a precipitous drop in the price of cane: they preferred no product to a possible loss of control to the workers. In Senegal, Franke and Chasin (1980) have documented the ways in which French control over land, and demand for the cash crop peanuts, destroyed subsistence production and the traditional symbiosis between farmers and herders.

All these cases illustrate how the total amount of food grown in any developing country, and global food production overall, are affected by land tenure. The specific impacts, in turn, of land tenure and associated crop choices on household and individual hunger depend on the relative prices of cash versus food crops, and on who benefits from cash-crop revenues. Additional factors are, on large holdings, whether workers are paid enough and food is plentiful and cheap enough to ensure a decent living; and on smaller holdings, whether the net income from cash crops more than compensates for the costs of foods that are no longer home-grown.

Crop choices and hunger impacts also depend on who controls the income from cash crops – control that, in traditional societies, is tied to gender-based land tenure and labour exchange. In the Gambia, women refused to contribute labour to their husbands' potentially highly productive irrigated rice plots (in this case rice was a food crop sold for cash) because they would not control the income, whereas they controlled food that they grew on their own lands (Jones 1983). A 20-year perspective on Nigerian peri-urban agriculture has shown that female cultivators, drawing on kinship-based land rights, have developed an unanticipated niche that supplies greater Ibadan with roots, tubers, fruits, and vegetables (Guyer 1995). In Kenya, non-governmental organizations (NGOs) and the FAO's International Plant Genetic Resources Institute (IPGRI) have designed pro-grammes to promote the production of indigenous food species for home consumption or market sales. Gardening everywhere is being encouraged as a way to increase food and fodder for internal markets and to improve household income and nutrition. Local gardening is also a way of conserving indigenous species in the environment.

Crop choices and production practices in much of Africa are changing in response to greater individualization of land holdings and wage labour but, as will be suggested further below, the impacts of such changes on food supply and household food security are pre-dictably mixed, since the circumstances are so variable.

Whether the context is cash or subsistence crops, an additional supply question is whether larger or smaller holdings are more pro-ductive or efficient. Wealthier landholders are more able to invest in agriculture – to assume the risks of new agricultural technologies and the recurrent costs of seeds, fertilizers, machinery, and labour. They may enjoy also superior access to credit and economies of scale in the purchase of inputs and in control over the prices for their products. There is no question that the early adopters of GR technologies were wealthier landowners who were able to absorb the risks and enjoyed major benefits. They became wealthier also by absorbing the small-holdings of neighbours who could not compete in the new productive environment. However, it is questionable whether production per unit land generally is higher on larger holdings, because smallholders, given the means, may invest labour and other inputs more carefully and achieve even higher outputs per unit area than their wealthier neighbours. Equitable or fair access to credit, crop insurance, inputs, and markets may remove most economies of scale. But under mod-ernizing agricultural conditions in much of the world, such conditions are hard to meet. Cooperative ownership and cultivation is one way that the possible disadvantages of smallholdings can be resolved; but, again, the evidence is mixed on whether larger communal or smaller individual holdings are more productive and efficient: so many other sociocultural and political economic factors besides landholding are involved in explaining why productivity is low on a Mexican ejido cotton cooperative or high on an Israeli citrus kibbutz.

In summary, the evidence on the ways in which land tenure influences agricultural investments and agricultural sustainability is mixed. Predictably, throughout the developing world, poverty and insufficient access to land result in unsustainable practices, including reduction of fallow, that lead to soil and water degradation, land exhaustion, and plummeting productivity. Farmers who lack resources to protect or improve land and water supplies have been blamed for soil erosion, desertification, and other ills (especially in SSA) and for deforestation and diminishing ecological resources and biodiversity in Asia and Latin America. Those working but not controlling the land can be expected to select the easiest or cheapest, rather than the most sustainable, cultivation practices. Morvaridi (1995) found that contract farmers in Cyprus used cultivation methods that were optimal only in the short run; because they did not own the land, they would not suffer the costs of long-run degradation. Conversely, extremely plentiful access to land can also discourage conservation: for example, extensive holdings in the Sudan have been tied to unsustainable agricultural methods that mine soil nutrients; after reaping initial profits, large landowners move on to exhaust additional areas. Whether owners deem it economic to maintain soil and water resources depends also on the conditions and costs of labour supply. Communally maintained terracing and waterways are falling into disrepair in countries such as the Philippines, where labour sees greater economic opportunities outside agriculture. Thus, land and labour constraints on productivity are closely tied, particularly under conditions of economic modernization and marginalization.

Labour

The amount of land that can be sown and harvested is, clearly, tied to available and affordable labour supply. Planting and harvesting are both activities that require far more labour than the rest of the agricultural cycle. In communities where these activities are shared, productivity on individual plots may be greater than if families had to provide all the labour that they could not afford to hire. Communal farming, although no longer common, provides some of the same advantages.

Where greater integration into the market economy disrupts traditional labour exchange, production may fall, as shown in Gudeman's classic study of a Panamanian village (Gudeman 1978). The reduction of patronage ties, such as in South Asian villages that have adopted GR technologies, may also produce labour bottlenecks that affect harvests. In many parts of SSA, modern cropping programmes fail where men control most of the land, technology, and proceeds but women are supposed to do much of the work, especially weeding. In Kenya, the increase in crop yield resulting from weeding was 56 per cent in female-headed households, but only 15 per cent in male-headed households; this led researchers to hypothesize that women do a less thorough job of weeding where they do not expect to control the benefits (Gittinger et al. 1990).

High labour costs may discourage extra hand cultivation and marginally lower outputs. But low agricultural wages discourage participation in the agricultural economy, where industrial or other opportunities exist. Very small household plots that cannot provide sufficient food and income push workers off the farm in search of income and can cause bottlenecks at planting and harvest times that lower food production. In Mexico, careful research into maize varieties and associated agricultural packages that would benefit small farmers proved less attractive and raised maize production less than anticipated; workers still could earn more off-farm, so abandoned farming. Scarcity of labour more than land is also a major constraint on production in much of Africa, where larger land areas since colonial times have experienced labour bottlenecks, as men were drawn off to work in the mines or to do other waged work and left women to clear, plant, and weed, with peak agricultural labour demands during the hungry season (Richards 1939). In such contexts, the problem of hunger is linked to underproduction in a vicious cycle.

Dietary preferences
An entire class of sociocultural issues related to food shortage have to do with consumption patterns and preferences. It is easy to think of these as relatively unimportant, because a preference for maize over sorghum in a food-short region is unimportant relative to total calorie availability. However, food preferences are one set of factors that determine what foods are grown and whether farmers, as in drought-prone SSA, sow and harvest drought-tolerant sorghum or sow a riskier maize crop that totally fails in drier seasons. The World Bank has identified overconsumption of wheat and rice as a key contributory factor to the African agricultural crisis: imports of these grains have soared over the last two decades to the detriment of local

production of other staple crops. Wheat and rice can both be grown in most African countries but only at costs far greater than the price of imports. Whether tastes for these imports grew in an era of economic prosperity, as was the case during the Nigerian oil boom years (Smith 1991), or as a result of dearth relieved by food aid, dependence on imports persists and has created a mismatch between economically feasible local production possibilities and consumer demand (Nwomonoh 1991). Burkina Faso, which was severely affected by the Sahelian drought of 1968–1974 and again by drought in the early 1980s, imported 94 per cent of its grain as wheat from 1966 to 1970. Wheat still constituted 52 per cent of grain imports during the first half of the 1980s, although the difference was made up by the traditional grains maize and sorghum (Barkin et al. 1990). It is not clear to what extent the continuing preference for imported wheat interferes with the country achieving food self-sufficiency during non-drought years; land, labour, access to technology, and income are probably more important factors.

Political and economic factors

Sociocultural factors influencing tastes and land or labour allocations are closely tied to political-economic forces, especially government policies and market conditions. This section considers other causes of food shortage that are tied to governments and markets – insufficient incentives for production, trade and import constraints, structural adjustment, and food aid. Political and economic factors related to conflict are dealt with in chapter 6.

Insufficient incentives for food production
Government initiatives to change consumption patterns out of economic self-interest are usually ineffective: Nigeria officially stopped rice imports in the mid-1980s in order to save foreign exchange, only to find that, by the end of the decade, rice consumption was still at two-thirds its previous level, owing to illicit re-exports of rice from Benin (Spencer et al. 1989, as cited in Reardon 1993). Efforts to protect local markets from inexpensive foreign grains (including cheaper products from neighbouring countries) are impeded by black market leakage that also distorts the food-availability situations in both donor and recipient countries. Government production and marketing-board policies, by contrast, very much influence what

farmers grow. In Kenya, government crop-breeding research, extension, and grain marketing in the 1980s focused on and successfully encouraged the production of maize, not sorghum; and in Tanzania, government crop insurance encouraged farmers in drought-prone areas to assume the greater risk and grow the less drought-tolerant (but, in a good year, more profitable) maize (Louis Putterman, personal communication 1995). Overall, relative crop prices influence what is grown, sold, or later consumed and thus influence food security at the national and household levels.

CASH-CROP VERSUS FOOD-CROP PROMOTIONS. Cash-crop promotions, by governments seeking to increase export earnings, may discourage production of food crops for local consumption through price, tax, and marketing structures. Some governments, as in Kenyan and Tanzanian promotions of tea and coffee, penalize farmers who wish to hedge their bets and maintain some subsistence production alongside cash crops, whose prices are outside the farmer's control. Others, as in the Mexican case cited above, provide incentives in the form of credits or crop insurance to grow particular cash crops, such as sorghum. Commercial export crops also expand relative to food crops where they enjoy the benefits of agricultural research and development, as well as priority access to critical inputs such as fertilizer (Hendry 1988). Where more resources are devoted to coffee than to millet, food availability may decline even while agriculture is modernizing, as was the case in Rwanda. Similar declines are reported where lands that could have produced basic food crops are shifted instead to more profitable livestock, forage, or animal feed (Barkin et al. 1990).

Export production can improve food availability for an individual country, if export earnings purchase more food than might otherwise have been grown. Islam (1994) demonstrated that the majority of countries that had expanded non-food production also experienced an increase in aggregate food supply. But countries that are dependent on raw-materials exports are often severely affected by even moderate shifts in world demand/prices of their products (Sheahan 1987). In addition, diversion of prime rice lands into higher-volume fruits and vegetables may account in part for the plateauing of the Asian GR in recent years.

Production incentives for crops are also limited if surpluses cannot be easily marketed. The US National Academy of Sciences (1986) noted that, in Africa, more intensive production systems tend to be located near railroad lines; in other areas, deteriorating transportation systems have discouraged remote agriculturists from responding to price increases for their products.

PRICE CAPS ON FOOD CROPS. Rural production is, however, more constrained overall by low food prices than by inability to respond to favourable prices. A large number of countries have governmental policies capping the prices of basic foodstuffs. These cheap food policies work primarily to the advantage of urban residents but discourage investments in the agricultural sector. Price ceilings on agricultural goods depress basic food production because rural producers have less incentive to grow food crops, farm larger areas, or intensify their production methods when the rate of return for their efforts is limited. Underpricing of agricultural products on the domestic market has been linked to slow rates of adoption of new agricultural technologies in a number of countries (UNICEF 1988).

Low food prices benefit urban dwellers and manufacturers who desire to keep wages low. Urbanites typically have less access to food through non-market channels than their rural counterparts and, more importantly, they are in a better position to pressure governments into protecting their interests. Even though the majority who are poor lack political power, manufacturers who pay urban wages put pressure on governments to keep urban prices low so that they can keep costs down and compete more effectively in internal and external markets.

In addition, in many countries, peasant producers buy and sell grain on a small scale throughout the year and therefore have conflicting needs as both producers and consumers (de Alcántara 1992). This is particularly true when landholdings are not large enough to meet household food needs, given the expense of agricultural inputs. Cheap food policies may receive political support even from the rural dwellers who would benefit most directly from their elimination.

Even without price ceilings, imported grain may be cheaper than locally produced grain if it is purchased from countries such as the United States that have more efficient, larger-scale production methods and that also subsidize production. Similarly, food aid – even if given only in crisis situations – may remove local incentives to produce surplus because local producers know that emergency carry-over stocks are available internationally (Brown and Kane 1994).

Local currency overvaluation also skews internal terms of trade in favour of urban dwellers since it renders imports artificially cheap, and imports drive down prices for domestic produce. The Nigerian naira was so overvalued during the oil boom that imported food was several times cheaper than locally produced food; Smith (1991) described domestic food production under these conditions as "almost irrational."

Higher prices for agriculturists in most cases increase aggregate food supply and contribute to food self-sufficiency. After years meeting its food needs by relying on lower-cost imports, the Belizean government provided incentives to agriculturists that offset the effects of controlled urban food prices; in 1981, Belize became self-sufficient in production of staple foods (Moberg 1992). However, the national marketing board operated at a loss because higher producer prices were not translated into higher consumer prices. Later, when government spending was limited by structural adjustment, the producers' price incentives were removed and the country again became a net importer of food.

OPPORTUNITY COSTS AND FOOD PRODUCTION. An additional consideration is that income from food crops must also be at a high enough level to meet opportunity costs of producing food rather than other cash crops or trade or wage goods. As consumers in the developing world become more integrated into the world economy they need more cash to purchase goods that they now desire but cannot produce themselves. Migration out of rural areas – either of entire families or, more commonly, of individuals – is often a temporary or repetitive strategy to earn cash. The same factors that create one-time need for urban employment often re-create it: patterns of circular migration between cities and the countryside are often repeated year after year. In sparsely populated rural areas, especially in sub-Saharan Africa, this creates a shortage of agricultural labour and a high dependency ratio. Older people and young children often remain in rural areas while those at prime productive economic ages migrate. Households have little incentive to maximize food production if their needs are better met by participation in the cash economy, particularly if some of their needs can *only* be met by participation in the cash economy. Shifts to less nutritious but less labour-intensive staple crops (especially cassava) have been tied to labour shortages (Benería and Sen 1986; Bukh 1979; FAO 1987; Huffman 1987; Protein–Calorie Advisory Group of the United Nations 1977; Tabatabai 1988; Thaman and Thomas 1985; Ware and Lucas 1988).

Even households that remain oriented toward subsistence agriculture usually need off-farm employment to generate the cash necessary to purchase agricultural inputs and additional food and non-food items. Labour shortage in agriculture has also emerged as a problem in more densely populated rural areas of Latin America, where intensive labour input is necessary to sustain or raise production. De Alcántara (1992) reported that, in Mexico, emigration by some household members in order to generate income for agricultural inputs increases both the need to rely on labour-saving herbicides and the use of hired day-labour. De Alcántara also noted the consequences of labour shortage for the rural community as a whole; households with high dependency ratios have very little labour to contribute to maintaining local irrigation networks and other public works that keep agriculture productive. They also have less incentive to adopt new labour-intensive technologies based on new seeds and chemical packages, if participation in manufacturing and service industries is more remunerative. Especially where farmers do not own land but must pay rent, net revenues after expenses can reduce incentives to grow food.

Producers are also less rewarded for their efforts if a portion of their crop must be paid to the landlord, as is common in sharecropping, and especially if they must repay debts assumed over the cultivation cycle immediately after the harvest, when grain prices are usually low. Even where rents are fixed, cultivators still do not have as much economic incentive to invest in methods that can raise production by retaining soil fertility from year to year. Thus, landholding, access to credit and markets, and relative income all affect production.

TAXATION POLICIES. State taxation policies also reduce incentives for rural agricultural production, since they transfer resources out of the rural sector. Appropriating revenue from the agricultural sector has proven to be one of the most successful short-run methods for increasing state revenue (Hinderink and Sterkenburg 1987). Production is taxed either directly or indirectly, in that many crops must be channelled through government marketing boards which, given low purchase prices, effectively appropriate a share of the produce. As the only legal consumer, marketing boards are in a position to set domestic prices that are typically held artificially low. If produce is sold at world market prices, the marketing board appropriates the difference. The effect of marketing boards is to depress producer prices, sometimes by as much as 85 per cent (Bates 1988).[3] Another indirect tax is licensing fees: farmers must pay for the right to cultivate or sell certain crops. All of these practices decrease producers' income. A number of studies conducted in the Philippines and reviewed by UNICEF (1988) concluded that government policies to support the farm sector were insufficient to overcome the negative effects of regulated pricing, government control of trade, export taxes, export quotas, and special levies. Government control of trade in certain Philippine commodities had much the same effect as marketing boards: potential profit was shifted from farmers to government agencies (UNICEF 1988).

Insufficient incentives for food production result from the combination of government policy and market forces. Together, they have created structural problems that interfere with food production and home-generated food supplies.

Trade and import constraints
A country's capacity to import food to compensate for production shortfalls is limited by its export earnings. However, it is overly simplistic to think of export earnings as a direct result of domestic productivity. World terms of trade effectively discriminate against products from developing countries. Although important steps toward trade liberalization have been made in the past decade, tariffs have been reduced to a greater extent on products from developed countries than those from developing countries. Under the General Agreement on Trade and Tariffs (GATT), tariffs are levied in proportion to the level of processing, a convention that exacerbates the inequality between already industrialized nations and those in earlier phases of the industrialization process. The General System of Preferences, which provides for the non-reciprocal reduction of tariffs on developing-country exports, has done little to compensate for this structural inequality because there are multiple individually negotiated preference schemes, many loopholes, and no legal guarantees that the provisions will be followed (Toton 1982).

Within countries, both food availability and revenues from export crops are limited by the ability of producers to market their crops. One of the most positive functions of marketing boards is to facilitate connections with remote rural areas and help develop infrastructure. However, the ability of centralized efforts to improve marketing can be limited by political will, timing of efforts, and available funds.

Although the Zambian government in 1985 pledged to haul all maize to safe storage before the onset of rains, the poor repair of roads – as well as the unavailability of grain bags, spare truck parts, and diesel fuel – made this impossible. Good (1986) observed that, even if the problems had been identified in time, government resources would have been insufficient to deal with them. Hence, Zambia was food short in a year with bumper harvests. In other countries, such as Belize, seasonally impassable roads are one of the reasons that urban dwellers rely on imported food (Moberg 1992).

When food is marketed between countries, transportation bottlenecks and lags can become significant issues. Some crops, particularly grains, are more durable, and less is lost if transportation is delayed at some point along the marketing route. For other crops, such as potatoes or vegetables, delays can mean seriously compromised quality or large losses.

Structural adjustment

Many of the political and economic constraints on production are related to heavy debt burdens in developing countries, which exacerbate their marginality and powerlessness to influence terms of trade in the world economy. In addition to the direct costs of financing debt, structural adjustment programmes designed by the World Bank and the International Monetary Fund (IMF) to promote debt repayment alter production relations in ways that can increase food shortage. Structural adjustment can have positive effects on food security in the long run. Restrictions on luxury imports can free foreign exchange for more necessary imports like fertilizer. Currency devaluation, restrictions on food imports, and lifting of food price controls may even increase local production, since some of the disincentives outlined above no longer apply. Food production has increased in some structurally adjusted economies (Meller 1992; Weeks 1995).

However, structural adjustment improves security via mechanisms that require a fairly extended time-frame. In the shorter run, financial austerity programmes associated with structural adjustment more often than not restrict food availability within affected countries. In India, attempts to reduce the government deficit led to decreased expenditures on rural roads, fertilizer subsidies, irrigation, agricultural extension services, agricultural research, and other rural infrastructure (Mukherjee 1994).

Structural adjustment policies that encourage exports of both food and non-food cash crops to meet external obligations can also create food shortage within regions. A structural adjustment process was implemented in Brazil in 1981; by 1983, per capita production of staple foods had declined by more than 15 per cent while per capita production of sugar cane increased by more than 35 per cent and cultivation of other exportables also expanded (Macedo 1988). Although basic food production rebounded somewhat in subsequent years, it did not grow as fast as export-oriented production, in spite of government programmes that attempted to expand vegetable gardening for local consumption (Macedo 1988). Similar effects have been documented in Peru in response to a more gradual adjustment programme from 1977 to 1985. Annual per capita food production fell by about 26 per cent during that period, and imports only partially compensated for the decline (Figueroa 1988). Thus, adjustment policies can have profound and long-lasting effects on the composition of agricultural production.

Food aid
Aside from these structural or economic issues, imports are also limited by the availability of humanitarian aid. Since there is no global food shortage, food for aid is clearly "available" in an absolute sense, but political agendas of both donor and recipient countries dictate that aid must serve other than strictly humanitarian ends. This finding is no longer shocking, in that US food donations have been made selectively on the basis of military, political, or economic importance at least since the 1970s and 1980s (e.g. Wallerstein 1980), and support to countries that are not of some strategic importance remains limited, although there has been some upsurge in humanitarian emergency assistance in the mid-1990s.

Food aid has successfully expanded commercial markets for producers in donor countries; in addition to fostering heavier dependence on imports, the availability of cheap, non-traditional grains helps change consumption patterns and thereby creates future demand for these grains (Toton 1982). Potentially receiving countries may have very different strategic importance when evaluated by political or military leaders than when evaluated by agribusiness executives. A country is most likely to receive priority for food aid when there is a clear humanitarian imperative, when donor governments are sympathetic to leaders currently in power in the needy country, *and* when future transfers through market channels are likely. The absence of any one of these factors can be limiting.

Interrelationships between causes of shortage

The environmental, sociocultural, and political/economic causes of food shortage are hardly independent. Even though inadequate fertilizer or water may place biological limitations on production, the main causes of disruption of fertilizer supplies and irrigation systems are economic; even though drought reduces food supply, it rarely leads to food shortage in the absence of armed conflict; even though consumer tastes and preferences are socially and culturally determined, they are heavily influenced by trade and aid.

Food production generally is more and more influenced by international market and policy trends as technology extends even into remote areas and as fewer agriculturists are self-sufficient (Jazairy et al. 1992). The terms of market integration are especially important: smaller producers may be protected against food shortage in cases of local food-crop failure, but they may be more vulnerable to food poverty overall. New agricultural technologies have been key factors allowing food production to keep pace with population growth on the global level, but local levels of food-grain production and incomes have become more variable among those using the technology (Chattopadhyay and Spitz 1987), and affordable food must be available to compensate for shortfalls.

There are some other downsides to increased agricultural productivity. Success in market production does not necessarily mean that production areas earn or produce enough to feed their populations. Vast increases in animal feed production and produce for urban markets in Mexico were accompanied by *decreased* production of basic foodstuffs. The "success" of these modern agricultural programmes attracted further financial and technical assistance, which reinforced the economic rationality of neglecting basic food production (Barkin et al. 1990). Similarly, favouring of soybeans relative to black beans increased productivity and Brazilian exports, but decreased beans as affordable and essential food for Brazilian producers and consumers. Specializing in export agriculture does not doom a region to food shortage but it does increase local or state-wide vulnerability to food shortage and shows that crop choices have important implications for world food supply.

The relationship between drought and famine

Some of the complex relationships between the causes of food shortage are best appreciated in the locations with prolonged drought.

They demonstrate that food shortage is not inevitable in regions that experience even major production shortfalls. There is much to be learned from cases where drought and other natural disasters did not end in famine, and particularly from developing countries that have succeeded in avoiding famine during lengthy drought.

The 1991/92 drought in Southern Africa, referred to as the "apocalypse drought" because of the magnitude of the problem, provides an unusually dramatic example of a large-scale natural disaster that resulted in very few deaths. Rains failed (or were late) across a wide region in 1991/92; the worst rainfall levels in over a century followed generally below-average rains across Southern Africa in 1989/90 and 1990/91. Grain yields in the ten states of the Southern African Development Community (SADC) were 56 per cent of normal[4] (Green 1993). Regional stockpiles were woefully inadequate to cope with the shortage. The drought placed 17–20 million people at risk of starvation. Yet there were no famine-related deaths reported, except in Mozambique where there was an ongoing civil war (Callihan et al. 1994).[5]

Famine preparedness and prompt response on the part of governments in the region to warning signs of famine are an important part of this success story. Even though regional stockpiles controlled by the SADC were insufficient to deal with the magnitude of the problem, the reserves were released onto the market early in the emergency, before food aid from other areas had arrived (Field 1995). Other interventions taken by governments in the region were far from novel but were implemented much earlier than similar strategies typically have been. Food imports and food aid, initiation or expansion of public works, and loans to agriculturists all addressed issues of supply and demand – rather than simply relief – early in the crisis (Field 1995). The government of Zimbabwe also pledged to purchase large quantities of grain before any donor aid had been committed; this proved to be a life-saving factor (Callihan et al. 1994).

Donors can be slow. Drought is nothing new in Southern Africa. Reports of low rainfall early in the 1991/92 growing season did not raise much alarm. There was some hope that later rains would salvage some reasonable crop yields, and there was little external donor perception of an emergency, despite a fairly well developed famine early warning system. Advances in early warning technology are of little use unless the warning signals are heeded (Buchanan-Smith et al. 1994). Before any external needs-assessment teams had arrived in the region, most of the SADC National Early Warning Units had already calculated initial food needs (Callihan et al. 1994). Nevertheless, it was 4–6 months before any donor aid reached Southern Africa in 1992. Relief food would have been even slower to arrive had it not been distributed through the SADC, which collected food in distribution centres even though it had not yet been determined where it ultimately was going (Callihan et al. 1994). Good rail, road, and communications infrastructure within the SADC facilitated delivery of food from the distribution centres.

Advance procuring of grain through market channels not only helped to provide food before aid arrived but also helped to avoid the precipitous price drops often associated with sudden arrival of vast quantities of food into drought-stricken regions. Grain prices thus remained relatively stable, protecting incomes of local farmers. Food also reached needy populations before they found it necessary to leave their homes. This greatly facilitated later rehabilitation efforts, since social and production systems were not disrupted. The advance commitment on the part of Southern African governments to import grain also helped prevent prices from being driven up by speculation, as has happened in other situations where crop failure has been accompanied by insufficient confidence in the ability of the government to import food (Ravallion 1987).

In addition, most food-distribution programmes were implemented through market channels, and rural works projects prevented collapse of rural markets during the crisis (Teklu 1994). Botswana did very well with a cash-for-work relief programme that was targeted to the poor by holding wages slightly below market rates (Callihan et al. 1994). The cash-for-work programmes were part of Botswana's Inter-Ministerial Drought Committee's ongoing relief activities (Quinn et al. 1988). Botswana has already done what the SADC is encouraging all of its member nations to do: it has built the expectation of drought into its budget, instead of treating it like a shock, and it has such programmes operating and ready to expand in case of drought.

Other countries in the region made use of both food-for-work and cash-for-work programmes. Almost all of the targeted food-distribution programmes were implemented through non-governmental organizations (NGOs) that had been operating in the affected communities prior to the drought. Resources came not only from the NGOs but also from proceeds from food sold through market channels. Maize subsidies were lifted in Zimbabwe and Zambia during the relief effort, to increase producer incentives at a time when large supplies of foreign maize would otherwise have driven prices down (Callihan et al. 1994). Malawi was the only country that relied on completely free distribution of food as part of its relief effort.

Although we have stressed the factors that prevented food aid from having detrimental effects on the region, the drought would almost certainly have led to famine in the absence of aid. The United States had record amounts of yellow corn on hand at the time that Southern Africa needed it most: about 12 million tons of grain were delivered in 1992 (Callihan et al. 1994). Some of the aid went through the World Food Programme and some of it was distributed through bilateral arrangements. The United States also provided US$112 million in non-food assistance, primarily in support of transportation and logistic coordination, agricultural rehabilitation and agricultural inputs, emergency water supplies, and health activities (Callihan et al. 1994). Importing was also easier during the drought, because the World Bank relaxed target dates for structural reform actions and made credit available.

Fortuitously, the bulk of grain available during the 1991/92 emergency in Southern Africa was the region's usual staple grain. Aid was then received without causing either temporary or longer-run shifts in local consumption patterns.

The lack of famine mortality, the lack of widespread social disruption, familiar relief foods, and distribution of food through market channels all made it easier for Southern Africa to recover from the disastrous agricultural conditions in 1991/92. Good weather in the following crop year (1992/93) was also critical, since it is unlikely that such a massive relief effort could have been sustained over time.

Other actions taken in response to the 1991/92 emergency made return to normal conditions quickly more plausible. The Sorghum and Millet Improvement Program of the International Crops Research Institute for the Semi-Arid Tropics (ICRISAT) in Matopos, Zimbabwe, provided (with funds from USAID) improved and tested varieties of drought-resistant small grains that matured earlier than the traditional varieties. These were approved for use in all of the SADC countries except Malawi – but even Malawi had a record agricultural harvest in 1993, in part due to improved maize seed that was distributed by an NGO (Callihan et al. 1994). Programmes had also expanded within the SADC to preserve cattle during times of drought, in order to help protect future livelihoods. These types of interventions were possible only because people in the region were not pushed into famine conditions under which they would have chosen short-run survival strategies over long-run subsistence strategies (Field 1995).

The experience of Southern Africa during the 1991/92 drought is not a complete success story. Mozambique fared less well than other Southern African countries, in part because donors were reluctant to send food aid that could be stolen by the Mozambican armed forces and not reach displaced people (Ayisi 1992). Production also did not rebound with the good rains in 1992/93 to the same extent as it did in neighbouring nations, largely owing to the ongoing civil war. Another, less severe, drought afflicted the region in 1994/95, and farmers who might otherwise have been able to cope were pushed into bankruptcy, since they were already in debt from the 1991/92 drought. Nevertheless, the experience during the worst drought in over a century clearly shows that drought does not have to lead to famine. The physical and biological causes of production shortfalls are in no way the sole determinants of food shortage. They must always be viewed against an institutional background dedicated to preventing and alleviating shortage.

Ecological and political aspects of food shortage in the 1990s

In evaluating the causes of food shortage, politics has been implicated more than the weather. This is because politicians shape the environment of response to ecological conditions. They also shape the trade-and-aid policies that determine whether households, regions, and countries produce enough food to provision themselves or have affordable terms for import and purchase. National politicians and policies also determine the extent to which regions and localities can retain or develop food self-reliance. Throughout much of the developing world, small farmers have capacities to improve production but lack certain access to land, moisture, seeds, and markets to make optimal use of that potential. They also lack access to basic services, such as health and education, that could improve their lives and prevent food shortage.

Since the 1990s, the international (UN) community has sponsored a number of century-end summit meetings to take stock of current resources and to plan for the future: these were the (UNICEF) World Summit for Children (1990), UNICEF–WHO Conference on Ending

Hidden Hunger (1991), International Conference on Nutrition (ICN, 1992), UN Conference on Environment and Development (UNCED, 1992), World Conference on Human Rights (1993), International Conference on Population and Development (1994), World Summit on Social Development (1994), Fourth World Conference on Women (1995), and World Food Summit (WFS, 1996). Almost all addressed two principal dimensions of food shortage and its prevention – the need for better mapping of hunger vulnerability, and the need for more stable political environments for food security. Although especially UNCED, the ICN, and the WFS addressed a plethora of additional technical, economic, social, and cultural issues surrounding food security now and into the twenty-first century, these two dimensions are probably the most significant for addressing local to global food-shortage problems. Implementation of the first is likely to be assisted by the momentum of political will generated by the various summits; implementation of the second is unlikely to be affected by international proclamations. In philosophical or humanitarian terms, few disagree that adequate food is a human right. But most continue to disagree over how to achieve universal food security in a world context divided by socio-economic inequalities, ethnic differences, and narrower country-level political interests. Biotechnological initiative that may break the "yield barrier," and adaptive research and extension to narrow the "yield gap" in basic foods, may help production keep up with population growth and prevent food shortage. But achieving food security for households and individuals remains a greater challenge.

Notes

1. There have been declines in carry-over stocks since 1993, but they are still above the level that the FAO considers necessary to maintain food security. Furthermore, all of the decline in stocks has occurred in developed countries as a part of pricing policy (Uvin 1996).
2. Higher fat consumption, accompanying improvements in household incomes, and access to food may mask the deteriorating nutritional status of poorer households, as both extremes are averaged in country-level consumption figures.
3. Marketing boards can have positive effects on producer prices when they act as producer cartels, but more often they act as monopsonies depressing prices (Krishna and Thursby 1992). Governments, especially in Africa, have widely used marketing boards to generate development funds.
4. They were 35 per cent of normal if Angola and Tanzania were excluded (Green 1993).
5. Undoubtedly, famine mortality would have been even higher in Mozambique if there were not a tentative peace during the drought which allowed relief shipments to reach the most affected (Callihan et al. 1994; Green 1993).

Works cited

ACC/SCN. 1993. *Second Report on the World Nutrition Situation; Volume II Country Trends, Methods and Statistics*. Geneva: Administrative Committee on Coordination, Subcommittee on Nutrition.

Albala-Bertrand, J. M. 1993. *Political Economy of Large Natural Disasters: With Special Reference to Developing Countries*. Oxford: Clarendon Press.

Ayisi, Ruth Ansah. 1992. "Mozambique: Drought and Desperation." *Africa Report* 37, No. 3: 33–35.

Barkin, David, Rosemary L. Batt, and Billie R. DeWalt. 1990. *Food Crops versus Feed Crops*. Boulder and London: Lynne Rienner.

Barraclaugh, S. 1989. *An End to Hunger?* London: Zed Books.

Bates, Robert H. 1988. "Governments and Agricultural Markets in Africa." In: Robert H. Bates, ed. *Toward a Political Economy of Development: A Rational Choice Perspective*. Berkeley: University of California Press, pp. 331–358.

Bender, W. H. 1994. "An End Use Analysis of Global Food Requirements." *Food Policy* 19: 381–395.

Benería, Lourdes, and Gita Sen. 1986. "Accumulation, Reproduction, and Women's Role in Economic Development: Boserup Revisited." In: Eleanor Leacock, Helen I. Safa, and contributors, eds. *Women's Work: Development and the Division of Labor by Gender*. South Hadley, Massachusetts: Bergin & Garvey, pp. 141–157.

Brown, Lester R., and Hal Kane. 1994. *Full House: Reassessing the Earth's Population Carrying Capacity*. The Worldwatch Environmental Alert Series, ed. Linda Starke. New York: W. W. Norton.

Buchanan-Smith, Margaret, Susanna Davies, and Celia Petty. 1994. "Food Security: Let Them Eat Information." *IDS Bulletin* 25, No. 2: 69–80.

Bukh, Jette. 1979. *The Village Woman in Ghana*. Copenhagen: Centre for Development Research.

Callihan, David M., John H. Eriksen, and Allison Butler Herrick. 1994. *Famine Averted: The United States Government Response to the 1991/92 Southern Africa Drought*. Management Systems International, Evaluation Synthesis Report Prepared for USAID/Bureau for Humanitarian Response. Washington, D.C.: Management Systems International.

Chattopadhyay, Boudhayan, and Pierre Spitz. 1987. "Introduction." In: Boudhayan Chattopadhyay and Pierre Spitz, eds. *Food Systems and Society in Eastern India: Selected Readings*. Geneva: United Nations Research Institute for Social Development, pp. 1–5.

Chen, Martha Alter. 1991. *Coping with Seasonality and Drought*. New Delhi: Sage.

de Alcántara, Cynthia Hewitt. 1992. *Economic Restructuring and Rural Subsistence in Mexico: Maize and the Crisis of the 1980s*. Discussion Paper 31. Geneva: United Nations Research Institute for Social Development.

Donahaye, E., and E. Messer. 1991. *Reduction in Grain Storage Losses of Small-Scale Farmers in Tropical Countries*. Research Report (RR-91-7), World Hunger Program. Providence, Rhode Island: Brown University.

FAO. 1987. "Women in African Food Production and Security." In: J. Price Gittinger, Joanne Leslie, and Caroline Hoisington, eds. *Food Policy: Integrating Supply, Distribution, and Consumption*. Baltimore: Johns Hopkins University Press, pp. 133–140.

————. 1992. *The State of Food and Agriculture*. Rome: Food and Agriculture Organization.

————. 1993. *Food Outlook*. Rome: Food and Agriculture Organization.

Field, John Osgood. 1995. "The Famine Process and the Phasing of Interventions." Paper prepared for the *Proceedings of the International Conference on Hunger* hosted by Glucksman Ireland House at New York University, New York, 19–20 May 1995.

Figueroa, Leonel. 1988. "Economic Adjustment and Development in Peru: Towards an Alternative Policy." In: Giovanni Andrea Cornia, Richard Jolly, and Frances Stewart, eds. *Adjustment with a Human Face: Volume II, Country Case Studies*. Oxford: Clarendon Press, pp. 156–183.

Foster, Phillips. 1992. *The World Food Problem*: Tackling the Cause of Undernutrition in the Third World. Boulder, Colorado: Lynne Rienner.

Franke, R., and B. Chasin. 1980. *Seeds of Famine: Ecological Destruction and the Development Dilemma in the West African Sahel*. Montclair, New Jersey: Allenheld, Osmun.

Gittinger, J. Price, Sidney Chernick, Nadine R. Horenstein, and Katrine Saito. 1990. "Household Food Security and the Role of Women." *World Bank Discussion Papers*, No. 96. Washington, D.C.: World Bank.

Good, Kenneth. 1986. "Systematic Agricultural Mismanagement: The 1985 'Bumper' Harvest in Zambia." *Journal of Modern African Studies* 24, No. 1: 257–284.

Grant, James P. 1995. *The State of the World's Children 1995*. New York: Oxford University Press for UNICEF.

Green, Reginald Herbold. 1993. "The Political Economy of Drought in Southern Africa." *Health Policy and Planning* 8, No. 3: 255–266.

Grigg, David. 1985. *The World Food Problem 1950–1980*. Oxford: Basil Blackwell.

Gudeman, Stephen. 1978. *The Demise of a Rural Economy: From Subsistence to Capitalism in a Latin American Village*. London: Routledge & Kegan Paul.

Guyer, J. 1995. Presentation in the Session "Land and Water Rights." Eighth Annual Hunger Research Briefing and Exchange, Brown University, Providence, Rhode Island, 5 April 1995.

Hendry, Peter. 1988. "Food and Population: Beyond Five Billion." *Population Bulletin* 43, No. 2.

Hinderink, J., and J. J. Sterkenburg. 1987. *Agricultural Commercialization and Government Policy in Africa*. London: KPI.

Huffman, Sandra J. 1987. "Women's Activities and Impacts on Child Nutrition." In: J. Price Gittinger, Joanne Leslie, and Caroline Hoisington, eds. *Food Policy: Integrating Supply, Distribution, and Consumption*. Baltimore: Johns Hopkins University Press, pp. 371–384.

Indonesian National IPM Program. 1991. *Farmers as Experts. The Indonesian National IPM Program*. Jakarta: Indonesian National IPM Program.

Islam, Nurul. 1994. "Commercialization of Agriculture and Food Security: Development Strategy and Trade Policy Issues." In: Joachim von Braun and Eileen Kennedy, eds. *Agricultural Commercialization, Economic Development, and Nutrition*. Baltimore: Johns Hopkins University Press, pp. 103–118.

Jacobsen, T., and R. M. Adams. 1955. "Salt and Silt in Ancient Mesopotamian Agriculture." *Science* 128: 1252–1258.

Jazairy, Idriss, Mohiuddin Alamgir, and Theresa Panuccio. 1992. *The State of World Rural Poverty: An Inquiry into Its Causes and Consequences*. New York: New York University Press.

Jones, Christine. 1983. "The SEMRY I Irrigated Rice Project." Paper presented to USAID, October 1983.

Krishna, Kala L., and Marie Thursby. 1992. "Optimal Policies and Marketing Board Objectives." *Journal of Development Economics* **38**: 1–15.

Lappe, Frances Moore. 1991. *Diet for a Small Planet*. 20th Anniversary Edition. New York: Ballantine Books.

———, and Joseph Collins. 1978. *Food First: Beyond the Myth of Food Scarcity*. New York: Ballantine Books.

Macedo, Roberto. 1988. "Brazilian Children and the Economic Crisis: The Evidence from the State of São Paulo." In: Giovanni Andrea Cornia, Richard Jolly, and Frances Stewart, eds. *Adjustment with a Human Face: Volume II, Country Case Studies*. Oxford: Clarendon Press, pp. 28–56.

Meller, Patricio. 1992. *Adjustment and Equity in Chile*. Development Centre Studies, Adjustment and Equity in Developing Countries, series ed. Christian Morrisson. Paris: OECD.

Mitchell, D. O., and M. D. Ingco. 1993. *The World Food Outlook*. Washington, D.C.: International Economics Department of the World Bank.

Moberg, Mark. 1992. "Structural Adjustment and Rural Development: Inferences from a Belizean Village." *Journal of Developing Areas* 27 (Oct.): 1–20.

Monteón, Michael. 1982. *Chile in the Nitrate Era: The Evolution of Economic Dependence, 1880–1930*. Madison: University of Wisconsin Press.

Morvaridi, Behrooz. 1995. "Contract Farming and Environmental Risk: The Case of Cyprus." *Journal of Peasant Studies* 23, No. 1: 30–45.

Mukherjee, Amitava. 1994. *Structural Adjustment Programme and Food Security: Hunger and Poverty in India*. Aldershot, England: Avebury.

National Academy of Sciences. 1986. *Population Growth and Economic Development: Policy Questions*. Washington, D.C.: National Academy Press.

Nwomonoh, Jonathon N. 1991. "Agricultural Policy and Production in Sub-Saharan Africa: Problems and Prospects." In: Valentine James, ed. *Urban and Rural Development in Third World Countries: Problems of Population in Developing Nations*. Jefferson, North Carolina: McFarland, pp. 38–48.

Protein–Calorie Advisory Group of the United Nations. 1977. *Women in Food Production, Food Handling and Nutrition: with Special Emphasis on Africa*. New York: United Nations.

Quinn, Victoria, Mark Cohen, John Mason, and B. N. Kgosidintsi. 1988. "Crisis-Proofing the Economy: The Response of Botswana to Economic Recession and Drought." In: Giovanni Andrea Cornia, Richard Jolly, and Frances Stewart, eds. *Adjustment with a Human Face: Volume II, Country Case Studies*. Oxford: Clarendon Press, pp. 3–27.

Ravallion, Martin. 1987. *Markets and Famines*. Oxford: Clarendon Press.

Reardon, Thomas. 1993. "Cereals Demand in the Sahel and Potential Impacts of Regional Cereals Protection." *World Development* 21, No. 11: 17–35.

Richards, A. 1939. *Land, Labour, and Diet in Northern Rhodesia. An Economic Study of the Bemba Tribe*. London: Routledge.

Sen, Amartya K. 1981. *Poverty and Famines: An Essay on Entitlement and Deprivation*. Oxford: Clarendon Press.

Sheahan, John. 1987. *Patterns of Development in Latin America*. Princeton, New Jersey: Princeton University Press.

Smith, Bamijoko. 1991. "The Impact of Structural Adjustment Policies on Agricultural Transformation and Poverty Alleviation in Africa." In: Valentine James, ed. *Urban and Rural Development in Third World Countries: Problems of Population in Developing Nations*. Jefferson, North Carolina: McFarland, pp. 22–37.

Tabatabai, Hamid. 1988. "Agricultural Decline and Access to Food in Ghana." *International Labour Review* 127, No. 6: 703–734.

Teklu, Tesfaye. 1994. "The Prevention and Mitigation of Famine: Policy Lessons from Botswana and Sudan." *Disasters* 18, No. 1: 35–47.

Thaman, Randolph R., and Pamela M. Thomas. 1985. "Cassava and Change in Pacific Island Food Systems." In: Dorothy J. Cattle and Karl H. Schwerin, eds. *Food Energy in Tropical Ecosystems*. New York: Gordon and Breach, pp. 189–223.

Toma, Ramses B., L. T. Fansler, and M. T. Knipe. 1991. "World Food Shortage: The Third Dimension." In: Valentine James, ed. *Urban and Rural Development in Third World Countries: Problems of Population in Developing Nations*. Jefferson, North Carolina: McFarland, pp. 61–66.

Toton, Suzanne C. 1982. *World Hunger: The Responsibility of Christian Education*. Maryknoll, New York: Orbis Books.

UNCTAD Secretariat, in cooperation with S. K. Mukherjee. 1985. *Fertilizer Supplies for Developing Countries: Issues in the Transfer and Development of Technology*. New York: United Nations.

UNDP. 1994. *Human Development Report 1994*. New York: Oxford University Press.

UNICEF. 1988. "Redirecting Adjustment Programmes toward Growth and the Protection of the Poor: The Philippine Case." In: Giovanni Andrea Cornia, Richard Jolly, and Frances Stewart, eds. *Adjustment with a Human Face: Volume II, Country Case Studies*. Oxford: Clarendon Press, pp. 184–217.

Uvin, Peter. 1994. "The State of World Hunger." *Nutrition Reviews* 52, No. 5: 151–161.

———. 1996. "The State of World Hunger." In: Ellen Messer and Peter Uvin, eds. *The Hunger Report: 1995*. Amsterdam: Gordon and Breach, pp. 1–17.

Wallerstein, Mitchel B. 1980. *Food for War–Food for Peace*. Cambridge, Massachusetts: MIT Press.

Ware, Helen, and David Lucas. 1988. "Women Left Behind, the Changing Division of Labor and its Effect on Agricultural Production." IUSSP Conference in Dakar, Senegal.

Weeks, John, ed. 1995. *Structural Adjustment and the Agricultural Sector in Latin America and the Caribbean*. New York: St. Martin's Press.

Wisner, Robert N., and Weiping Wang. 1990. *World Food Trade and U.S. Agriculture, 1960–1989: Changing the Rules of Trade*. Tenth edition. Ames, Iowa: Midwest Agribusiness Trade Research and Information Center.

Wolf, E. 1969. *Peasant Wars of the Twentieth Century*. New York: Harper and Row.

Woodham-Smith, C. 1962. *The Great Hunger, Ireland 1845–9*. New York, Harper and Row.

World Bank. 1992. *World Development Report 1992*. Washington D.C.: The World Bank.

4

Food poverty

Laurie F. DeRose

Food poverty here refers to household-level hunger. Households in food poverty do not have enough food to meet the energy and nutrient needs of all of their members. Depending on patterns of intra-household distribution, at least one member of a food-poor household is always hungry but, potentially, all members are.

This chapter first explores the causes of food poverty. The main issues in the international distribution of food are considered first, but more attention is given to the national distribution of food and why household entitlement to food sometimes fails. It then reviews the evidence for the distribution of food poverty across the world, types of evidence used to measure food poverty, and trends in the incidence of food poverty over time. The chapter then turns to the more piecemeal evidence available on *which* households within regions are the most likely to be affected by food poverty, evidence that provides further insight into how households succeed or fail in providing food for their members. To emphasize the importance of non-market access to food in protecting households from hunger, a case study of food-sharing networks is included. The chapter concludes with recommendations for reducing food poverty.

Causes of food poverty

Some households live under conditions of chronic or seasonal food poverty. Other households are pushed into food poverty because of changes in area food availability and/or in their own ability to secure entitlement to food.

Food shortage

Food availability in a region is one of the key determinants of the existence and extent of food poverty. In food-short regions, at least some households are food poor. But widespread food poverty persists in the absence of shortage, and many households escape food poverty despite severe food shortage.

Given no shortage of food on the global level, all incidence of food poverty can be attributed to maldistribution rather than underproduction. "Distribution" in this context includes transportation and storage, as well as production patterns and crop choices; it is not simply a matter of shuffling around existing food.

Reducing food shortage at national and sub-national levels is an important tool for reducing food poverty, but not simply because lack of shortage eliminates the necessity of food poverty. Productive and distributive mechanisms – not just food availability – change when there is food shortage. Famines, embargoes, and structural adjustment all cause shifts in the conditions of exchange that lead to entitlement failure (Ravallion 1987). Changes in food production affect at-risk households primarily through changes in income and prices, rather than as a direct result of food supply. Famine may also cause smallholders ordinarily subsisting on the margin to destitute themselves by selling land and other assets – acts that permanently shift the power and social structure of a society.

A special case of food shortage is violent conflict that reduces food availability and changes patterns of food distribution in affected countries. Food imports during times of violence are often restricted by embargoes. During both international and intranational conflict, governments put a high priority on provisioning the military, which tends to decrease civilian access to food. Although it is theoretically possible for local food production to increase enough to offset the food deficit caused by embargoes and diversion of existing supplies to the military, this usually does not happen quickly enough to avoid increased poverty. It is much more common for internal food production to decrease, because land has been abandoned and livestock sold by agriculturists seeking to avoid being plundered (Tschirley and Weber 1994). It is also quite difficult to expand production when economic and human resources are being devoted to the conflict.

Also, different households are likely to suffer from food poverty in times of embargoes and other trade restrictions. Although many of those ordinarily food poor may still suffer, some poor households will benefit from having members in the military and, even if there are no direct benefits, resources then do not have to be shared as many ways. In addition, warfare may increase certain kinds of production, creating new employment and income. However, in most recent conflict situations there are many more losers than beneficiaries, because of destruction, looting, and political control of food distribution. When the share of marketed food goes down, the resources required to obtain it can be prohibitive.

Commerce restrictions also have effects on food poverty that do not operate through shortage. Households whose livelihoods depend on wages from industries that specialize in export goods may be especially vulnerable to food poverty if embargoes lead to unemployment or underemployment for workers in those industries. A fuller discussion of the effects of employment on food poverty follows in the section on entitlements.

Social displacement

People driven across international borders as a result of war or civil strife are refugees. The most fortunate of refugees may be able to contact family members who migrated in less stressful times, but most leave behind possessions, sources of income, and social ties. Abrupt social displacement removes most customary sources of entitlement to food and for many, charitable distributions are the only buffers between them and starvation. Food insecurity among refugee populations is a concern of the United Nations and non-governmental organizations (NGOs), who raise money, food, and resources to relieve poverty and hunger throughout the world.

The situation of refugees highlights the well-known relationship between hunger and infection. Mortality in refugee camps is very high, but little is attributed exclusively to hunger. Concentration of people in refugee camps brings diseases from a wide range of locations, and these diseases spread rapidly among people already weakened by hunger (Seaman 1993). Those whose immunity is compromised by poor food intake are often unable to withstand infections that would not be life threatening under ordinary circumstances.

Macroeconomic policies

Government spending and poverty-alleviation efforts influence economic activity, employment, incomes, and household access to food. Exchange rates, balance of trade, debt repayment, and other financial institutions all provide an environment that conditions what economic activities households pursue and whether food is available and affordable. Many countries, prior to the oil crisis of the 1970s, pursued economic policies that relied heavily on debt spending and provided hefty food subsidies and government-sponsored health care for the poor. As debt became an ever-greater burden, the international financial community insisted that governments "adjust" their spending and restructure public enterprise. The set of policies developed to enforce greater fiscal responsibility are called "structural adjustment" or "adjustment" policies. Although the goal of structural adjustment is to build a healthier economy for the long run, the associated policies that cut social welfare spending, readjust exchange rates downward, and insist on greater investment in exports, including export crops, have been blamed for much of the food poverty that currently afflicts the countries affected.

Structural adjustment

Structural-adjustment policies have been negotiated between international financial institutions – primarily the World Bank and the International Monetary Fund (IMF) – and a large number of developing countries. These allow debt-repayment schedules to be redrawn but they also impose conditions that affect the structure of trade and government spending. The purpose of these is to restructure both production incentives and consumption patterns, so that there is a better match between a country's resources and its economic activities. If structural adjustment achieved all of its goals, adjusted countries would demonstrate sustained economic growth that would allow them to repay their debts and remain out of debt in the future.

The process of structural adjustment changes national food availability because it typically involves currency devaluation, which increases the real prices of imported food. It also changes the price of food and other goods relative to the price of labour; this has important implications for the ability of households to secure access to food. Even households that may benefit from structural adjustment in the longer run are likely to have difficulty securing access to food during rapidly changing social and economic conditions.

External debt and debt financing are important constraints on the ability of nations both to import food and to invest in their own agricultural sectors to enhance future production. The size of the debt burden in developing nations can be better appreciated by comparing the size of the national debt with gross national product (GNP);

in 1992 the less-developed countries as a whole produced only about three times as much as they owed. In Latin America and the Caribbean, debt was 38.1 per cent of GNP, and in sub-Saharan Africa it was 88.2 per cent of GNP (World Bank 1994). It is not realistic to believe that countries can expand agricultural production if huge shares of their economic surplus are being spent on debt service and imports.

Unfortunately, even if structural-adjustment programmes would be tremendously successful in the long run, their short-term effects are often devastating. One of the most common macroeconomic policy changes made by adjusting countries is the devaluation of foreign exchange rates. Having an overvalued currency keeps imports artificially cheap, and, after devaluation, less food can be imported, given the same amount of foreign exchange. This particular cause of food shortage is most likely to lead to food poverty for the urban poor. Urban dwellers usually have less flexibility and resources to produce their own food and are therefore likely to rely on markets. Since devaluation is often accompanied by wage freezes in both the private and the public sectors, food prices rise while incomes do not.

Domestic export industries tend to expand with devaluation (because the same volume of exports earns more in the local currency), but the time-lag between devaluation and employment expansion is usually substantial, especially under the conditions of recession that accompany the adoption of structural-adjustment policies. Recession and adjustment are linked for two main reasons. First, recession usually precedes adjustment: countries often agree to the terms of adjustment policies because stagnation in their economies gives them little hope of repaying debt on normal, commercial terms. Second, potential to expand production is limited because debt finance and repayment – even on renegotiated terms – consume surplus that could have been reinvested in the economy.

Inflation aggravates the plight of households in adjusting countries. When faced with both higher food prices and higher prices for other necessary goods, these households must trade off their limited resources. Urban households that have lost formal employment, or who find their income inadequate in the face of inflating prices, often compensate by expanding informal-sector activities, but the profitability of these is especially limited during times of recession. Even though structural adjustment hits the urban poor harder than most rural dwellers, higher prices for agricultural inputs also have severe effects on rural dwellers. In Mexico, growing maize on plots already conditioned to the use of herbicides and fertilizer became unafford-able to many farmers under structural adjustment (Collier 1990).

Overall, structural-adjustment programmes affect the entire econ-omy and decrease private incomes at all levels, but poorer house-holds are disproportionately disadvantaged (Macedo 1988). Even in countries where income per capita has grown significantly, the income-distribution effects of adjustment contribute to income inequality (Serageldin 1990) and increase the likelihood that more households will be in food poverty. Anti-poverty and welfare programmes that directly address the health and food needs of the most disadvantaged can help lessen the pain of structural adjustment, but the poor are still usually left worse off both relatively and absolutely.

Social dimensions of adjustment
The World Bank has tried to limit the impact of adjustment on income distribution. Their Social Dimensions of Adjustment project and other poverty-alleviation programmes include interventions intended to increase access to employment and food for the urban poor and access to land and credit for the rural poor. Public employ-ment schemes and food-for-work programmes have the advantage of targeting scarce resources more effectively to poor households than do direct food-supplementation programmes. In Senegal, the gov-ernment has sponsored retraining and rural-resettlement schemes for laid-off civil servants and laid-off workers from the manufacturing sector (Serageldin 1990). Such capacity-building programmes are critical in preventing adjustment from miring greater numbers in food poverty. Interventions that relocate underemployed urban workers into rural areas promote agriculture and potentially help reduce the chances of food shortage in adjusting countries.

Social Dimensions of Adjustment programmes have been added to adjustment schemes to compensate in part for health care and nutrition programmes that could not keep up with rising demand for services while government expenditures on them was limited by the adjustment package. Programmes that seek to mitigate the social costs of adjustment are challenged by limited financing, limited knowledge of the most vulnerable groups, and limited capacity to target interventions. These difficulties help explain why they are not always successful. The rapid pace of social and economic change under structural adjustment further complicates these problems. Food hand-outs are more difficult to target to the poor than food-for-work schemes, which tend to attract only those who do not have other viable employment options. However, if interventions do not reach the poor promptly, free food distribution may have to precede work-based programmes because the poor will need improved nutrition before they are healthy enough to work.

Entitlement failure of households

The use of the concept of entitlements for understanding hunger has been popularized by the work of Amartya Sen (examples include Drèze and Sen 1990; Sen 1981a, 1981b). Own production, stored wealth, employment, kinship, and government transfers are all possible sources of food entitlement. Sen distinguished among endowments (e.g. land), exchange (e.g. wage), and social-security entitlements. While other approaches recognize that access to food is as critical a determinant of household hunger as is total production, the entitlement approach does not assume a fixed pattern of inequality in the distribution of food: instead, it focuses on how people acquire food. At low income levels, households whose entitlement to food comes from a single source are much more vulnerable to food poverty than those who have multiple sources of entitlement. Some sources of entitlement are also more stable than others. Diversification across and within food-entitlement categories limits risk of food poverty.

Opportunities for households to diversify risk are somewhat limited where all members typically reside in fairly close proximity to one another, so that labour market and other economic opportunities do not extend easily beyond the production patterns in their place of residence, particularly in rural areas. One way to transcend this limitation is by out-migration of individual members, who may no longer eat with the household on a regular basis but who retain important economic and affective ties. Migrant members who return to the household frequently, to visit, bring money, or contribute agricultural labour, are referred to in the demographic literature as "circular migrants." The contribution of remittances from circular and other migrants toward entitlements to food will be considered in greater detail below.

Access to land (resource-endowment entitlements)
Land, especially land ownership, is perhaps the most critical entitlement for preventing a household's food poverty in rural areas. In addition to providing food in ordinary times, access to land can safe-

guard against household hunger in situations where food supply is limited by non-environmental factors such as changes in food prices brought about by trade policy. It also provides an asset in protecting against food poverty and destitution if production is limited by factors such as widespread drought.

Land ownership is the most secure means of gaining access to land. Other arrangements, such as patron–client relationships, share-cropping, tenant farming, and use of communal lands also provide production-based entitlement to food, but are less reliable during times of crisis. Chen (1991) showed that, in Gujarat, those with insufficient land were customarily allowed to use private pastures and forest groves, but that these rights were withdrawn during drought.

The value of land for securing entitlement to food is further conditioned by labour availability, which a household must itself provide or otherwise purchase. Purchase-price controls on basic food crops limit earnings from sales of surpluses, pushing farmers toward greater production of non-food cash crops or off the farm into the urban sector. Both responses limit the amount of (particularly male) labour available for food production. The ability of women to sustain food production, where male labour has been diverted to other activities, has been limited by sheer time and energy constraints, as well as by less-frequent contacts with agricultural extension workers, the diversion of their labour to cash crops or other income-earning activities, and their numerous domestic and child-rearing responsibilities.

Additional evidence for how important access to land is for the nutritional status of rural households is reviewed below in the section on within-rural variation in the distribution of food poverty.

Employment (exchange entitlements)
Most labour-market activities (self-employment or employee) are remunerated in cash, which is then exchanged for food. Some forms of employment (especially in agriculture) involve transfer of food directly to employees. Even households engaged primarily in subsistence agriculture frequently have at least one member who is employed off the family farm; this is an important risk-avoidance strategy.

Food entitlements are closely tied to jobs and wage rates, which is why employment statistics are critical indicators of food poverty. Formal-sector jobs in developing economies are difficult to secure; loss of such a job may cause a dramatic drop in family income, since finding other employment with the same pay rate may be a lengthy or impossible process. Employment in informal economic activities presents different challenges, since many of those employed in the informal service sector, cottage industry, and marketing are chronically or sporadically underemployed, even if they never face open unemployment. Compensation may be so pitiful that working even more than full time does not always garner enough income to ensure entitlement to food for all household members.

In crisis situations, successful government initiatives to prevent famine in cases of large-scale food-production shortfalls include employment creation; lost entitlements are re-created through wage-based government employment (Drèze and Sen 1990). These programmes allow food distribution to continue through normal economic channels and limit the social costs of widespread unemployment.

Food poverty persists in non-crisis situations and presents one of the key difficulties that developing countries face as they seek to modernize their production systems without increasing hunger. Modern production methods usually replace labour with capital and import the machinery from countries where labour is more expensive. The forces determining wages and employment levels in modern agriculture are different, but the net effect of modernization still is to limit employment-based entitlement to food. Modern crop varieties (e.g. hybrids, high-yielding varieties) that began to be introduced with the Green Revolution in the 1970s have expanded overall demand for agricultural labour. The yield from these new varieties depends heavily on labour-intensive transplanting, weeding, fertilizing, irrigating, and application of pesticides. Modern varieties of wheat and rice require 20–40 per cent more labour than traditional varieties (Mebrahtu et al. 1995). But population growth and in-migration into regions where agriculture has modernized have kept rural labour supply high and rural wages low (Mebrahtu et al. 1995). Mechanization in some cases has reduced rural employment, especially where governments subsidize imports of labour-saving machinery with the intent of increasing agricultural productivity (Mebrahtu et al. 1995). Resulting decreases in rural employment and/or wages can push rural households into food poverty.

All households that rely on employment-based entitlement to food are vulnerable to changes in the structure of production or the competitiveness of labour markets. Surplus labour that spills over from the agricultural to the industrial or service sectors is typically unskilled and untrained, and individual productivity may be limited by poor health and nutritional status. Those who remain unemployed or underemployed for a period of time find that they are less-effective employees and also earn less at self-employment. Under these constraints, households disadvantaged by low earning power at one point in time have little ability to improve their earning potential and need health and nutritional programmes to prevent their further deterioration into food poverty. These are not problems faced by those in more skilled positions or modern-sector industries.

Prices and wages

The degree of food security depends on prices as well as labour productivity and income. Although increased agricultural productivity usually leads to higher incomes and better food security among households that have access to modern inputs and methods, the food security of households that continue to use less-productive methods depends largely on the degree to which production expansion drives down food prices and on how much food they sell rather than buy. Small-scale farmers often consume a share of their own produce, but it is increasingly rare for household food needs to be met entirely by subsistence production. Where prices of other foods, such as legumes, increase dramatically relative to staple grains, some farmers cannot afford to purchase what they do not produce. Even households that are mostly food self-reliant find their food security compromised where lower food prices mean they have to sell a greater share of their own production to meet their non-food needs. More advantageously, higher agricultural production that lowers food prices improves the access to food in non-landed households.

Increases in the prices of essential non-food items, such as fuel and housing, also aggravate food poverty in low-income households, regardless of income source. Households may try to minimize the impacts of rising prices by shifting their consumption patterns, but lack of fuel poses an insurmountable barrier to food preparation.

Prices for all goods are influenced by exchange rates. Many developing countries overvalued exchange rates in an effort to make imports cheaper for their residents; it takes fewer pesos to buy a sack of wheat if the peso is overvalued. In the wake of the debt crisis, and with the widespread adoption of structural-adjustment programmes, fewer countries maintain overvalued currencies. Having imports available only at world-market prices in economies where the currency used to be overvalued means that the same sources of entitlement will not command the control over the same products.

Kinship (social-security entitlements)
Protecting households from sudden jolts and destitution under shifting economic conditions are the traditional (and increasingly non-local) sources of social security. Many households avoid hunger, in periods when their exchange entitlements to food fail, through kinship ties. These food-provisioning networks protect households from sudden drops in their own production and income but are less effective where economic conditions or environmental shocks affect food availability for most in the network. For example, a father who loses his tenant rights to cultivate land can rely on kin for food while he is seeking alternative employment, but if drought depresses all agricultural production, fewer resources are available to share within the kin network.

Kin networks nourish in multiple ways: customary rules of hospitality dictate that kin present at a meal be fed, and food is often sent home with visiting kin as parting gifts. Children may be fed by, or sent to live with, relatives who provide for their food and health needs (Desai 1992). In West Africa, child fosterage occurs in both crisis and non-crisis situations and it is common enough that such arrangements do not create unusual social obligations or even necessitate admitting that the sending family is unable to care for their child(ren) alone.

Kin networks also transfer cash – especially important where someone lives and works in another location. Among the poorest 10 per cent of households in Botswana, 25 per cent of household income is supplied by transfers from other households or family members living elsewhere (Quinn et al. 1988). The role and reliability of migrant remittances are discussed further below.

Kinship links may be created explicitly for the purpose of safeguarding access to food. Marriage ties and "fictive kin" arrangements extend food-sharing obligations and entitlements to non-blood relations. Even very poor families decrease their vulnerability to hunger by giving away food and other gifts in ways that create links to people who will help them in more desperate situations (Adams 1993). It is also customary for age mates in African societies to share food and labour with one another.

Such food-sharing obligations and benefits tend to shrink, however, as the total resources of a community drop. In Gujarat, India, Chen (1991) documented food sharing with a wide variety of caste neighbours when food was plentiful, but non-market exchanges were based primarily on kinship ties during lean times. In rural Africa, sociability declines along with food supply: people eat alone to avoid the obligation to share (Messer 1984).

Female headship in some situations also reduces food flows from kin. Households that are headed by women because the husband is a temporary migrant or lives with one of his other wives may be just as well integrated into kin networks as those who reside with their husbands. This is also likely to be true of female-headed households among matrilineal groups. However, if female headship represents a permanent separation of a woman from her husband or the father of her children, her household may lose the benefits of food sharing with his relatives. For example, divorced women in Ghana have little contact with their husbands' kin, while other women who do not live with their husbands typically live with (or very close to) co-wives, in-laws, and other patrikin (Lloyd and Brandon 1991). In other countries, such as Haiti, marital status matters less because food-sharing networks are entirely female.

Migrant remittances
Migration that reduces the numbers that need to be fed and/or increases potential income for food is a principal mechanism of risk aversion. Migrant family members, whether they circulate between areas or permanently change residence, give households access to remote labour markets where wages may be far higher, or at least fluctuate at different times. Disadvantages for those left at home in rural areas may include insufficient household labour to sustain home food production and the unreliability of migrant remittances. Many who migrate to urban areas fail to find formal-sector employment, and jobs in the tertiary sector may not earn enough surplus to remit back to the rest of the household. Rural households may even have to provide food for urban members while the latter are seeking employment, particularly where both food and fuel in urban areas are scarce and more expensive (Fuller et al. 1990; Goldscheider 1983).

Regularity of remittances varies and seems to be related to the frequency of return visits. Migrants who return home regularly may be more integrated into their households and feel more accountable. Additionally, the channels for sending money in developing countries are frequently undeveloped, and remittances may not be forthcoming unless the migrant or a trusted friend is personally travelling back to the area of origin. Even when other channels are used, large amounts

103

may not be risked: circular migrants from Mali to France tend to bring more money home when they visit than they send while they are away (Findley 1994).

Given its unreliability, income from migrants typically does not supplement household food budgets as much as would otherwise be expected. Few studies have distinguished source of income from type of income, but Kaiser and Dewey (1991) found that sporadic remittances were associated with decreased food quality and with retarded growth of preschool children in rural Mexico. Lump sums tend to be spent on consumer durables, such as roofing sheets or bicycles, which require significant savings to buy and may be the "target" for which migration was undertaken.

Having migrant household members may help in times of crisis, but the ability to migrate during a crisis is limited by poverty and the numbers similarly displaced and looking for work. Findley (1994) reported that Malians working overseas were expected to increase remittances in times of drought-induced crop failure, but that such long-range migration was difficult to launch in response to drought because of cost. During the 1983–1985 Malian drought there were significantly increased levels of internal migration, but this served primarily to reduce the number of members in rural households, rather than to generate additional income (Findley 1994).

Flawed government policies

Excessive taxation

Taxation poses another drain on household resources: when taxes rise, the ability of households to meet food and other needs falls. Higher taxes differ in some ways from other price rises, however. Taxes on luxury goods and income can be used to generate government revenue without burdening the poor, but other tax structures can be quite regressive, as is the case with a sales tax.

Taxes can be used to alter the structure of production, as where exporting industries are given tax breaks in order to increase their capacity to earn foreign exchange, or where taxes on rural producers force them to produce cash crops over subsistence crops. As reviewed in chapter 3, taxes on agriculture are favoured by governments, who privilege newly developing urban industries even though these reduce food-production incentives and affect household entitlements and access to food.

Taxation, additionally, is a mechanism by which governments redistribute wealth and food and has the potential to reduce food poverty. Nutritional supplementation programmes reach households not productive enough to be directly affected by a tax burden. Public health programmes reduce nutritional requirements because of the synergism between infection and disease; those that have been particularly effective in a wide variety of contexts include immunization, sanitation, and oral rehydration therapy. Government investments also expand job opportunities in both public and private sectors, thereby raising employment-based entitlement to food. Alternatively, poor investment decisions contribute to economic stagnation or promote capital-intensive industries that employ few workers. Many nutrition and health programmes fail to reach the neediest. In sum, taxation and tax-revenue spending in any particular country clearly influence production choices, household resources, and the distribution of food and health.

Insufficient government safety nets

Direct feeding, food supplementation, food stamps, and subsidies are all programmes designed to raise the real incomes and food consumption in households (Rogers 1995). Giving food directly to households improves intake, if money that would have been spent on food in the absence of the transfer is not spent instead on other goods. Providing households with more food than they were purchasing in the absence of the programme guarantees an improvement in income but is too costly to be practical. Instead, smaller transfers are targeted toward poor households in ways that will be most likely to increase food consumption, even though there may be some leakage.

Government safety nets function most effectively when they utilize existing markets to distribute food; common mechanisms include food stamps, ration shops, and specially subsidized foods (Kates 1996). It is difficult to reach households on a sustained basis with food–welfare programmes (particularly in rural areas), but changing social, economic, and environmental conditions continually re-create the need for short-term assistance as well as for programmes that create and diversify entitlements. Even for households whose entitlements are usually sufficient to avoid food poverty, government programmes may be necessary to cope with additional stress introduced by disease (Kates 1996).

Given the difficulty of designing and implementing interventions that will absolutely increase household food intake, such programmes are arguably most important as a relatively stable source of household entitlement to food. Even if children consume less at home if fed through school lunch or other direct-feeding programmes, their intake is less vulnerable to changes in family income than it is in the absence of such a programme. Even if direct feeding and other similar programmes do not have dramatic effects on intake in "normal" times, they may shield households from food poverty in times of crisis. Supplementary feeding has been shown to decrease the prevalence of both moderate and severe malnutrition in children; it was an important component of the Iringa nutrition programme in Tanzania, which succeeded despite being implemented during early stages of structural adjustment (Serageldin 1990). Supplementary-feeding programmes have also been highly successful in parts of India, including Tamil Nadu. Such programmes are often administered through existing health and education systems.

Kinds of data

Although the sources of entitlement failure are well understood in theory, identifying which households are suffering – or even the types of household or number of households that suffer – from food poverty is more difficult. Calculations of the extent of food poverty rely on estimates of household food availability relative to need and measures of absolute poverty.

Estimated numbers in absolute food poverty

The FAO and the World Bank regularly publish estimates of the numbers of chronically undernourished people. Their findings are based on national food availability and information about its distribution across households. Many issues related to data collection and comparability were described in chapter 2 of this volume. The implications of the slightly different methodologies used by the two institutions are described below in the section on trends. Importantly, both institutions base estimates of food poverty on the *distribution* of food and income rather than simply per capita supply versus availability or consumption versus expenditure. This attention to household command over food results in a picture of hunger that differs greatly from the regional food-availability estimates presented in

Table 4.1 **Proportions and numbers of chronically underfed by world region**

									Region
Underfed	Year	Sub-Saharan Africa	Near East and North Africa	Middle America	South America	South Asia	East Asia	China	All LDCs[a]
Proportion	1970	35	23	24	17	34	35	46	36
(%)	1975	37	17	20	15	34	32	40	33
	1980	36	10	15	12	30	22	22	26
	1990	37	5	14	13	24	17	16	20
Absolute	1970	94	32	21	32	255	101	406	942
numbers	1975	112	26	21	32	289	101	395	976
(millions)	1980	128	15	18	29	285	78	290	846
	1990	175	12	20	38	277	74	189	786

Source: Uvin (1994) as taken from ACC/SCN (1992: 105).
a. LDCs: less-developed countries.

chapter 3. Distribution-entitlement failures matter for hunger. Table 4.1 shows the numbers and percentages of people suffering from food poverty.

Although income data are notoriously difficult to collect, they are still less complicated than food-intake data; this is one of the reasons that estimates of numbers in absolute poverty are often used to estimate the numbers that are hungry. There is also a strong theoretical basis for this method: those who are among the poorest are also the least likely to be able to feed themselves and their families.

Despite the logical simplicity of this approach, non-market sources of entitlement, coupled with measurement error on incomes, could cause large discrepancies between the numbers in absolute poverty and numbers of households that are food poor. Fortunately, this appears not to be the case generally. FAO estimates of the numbers who are hungry correspond to estimates of numbers in absolute poverty, both in magnitude and in their direction of change over time. Changes in food poverty are estimated fairly accurately from changes in prevalence of absolute poverty. This generalization holds true across all areas of the developing world except East Asia, where the incidence of hunger is much higher than the incidence of poverty and where hunger declined between 1980 and 1990 even though the numbers in poverty did not change (Uvin 1994).

Trends in global food poverty

Worldwide trends in food poverty have been downward, despite rapid population growth in most of the developing world. Such trends are based on the most recent methodologies. Over the period from 1970 to 1990, the FAO adjusted several times its methodology for calculating the number of malnourished people, but the estimates were most commonly based on defining minimal food intake at 1.4 times the basal metabolic rate (BMR), or 40 per cent more calories than basal metabolic functions require. Intake of less than 1.2 BMR is considered inadequate, even for sedentary people, because even the most basic processes such as digestion require additional calories; 1.4 BMR allows for only minimal physical activity (WHO 1985). When the FAO recalculated estimates of hunger from 1970 to 1990 using a standard methodology, it selected a cut-off of 1.54 BMR, which allows for light physical activity.

Using this higher and more realistic cut-off produced hunger estimates for the recent past that were considerably higher than those reported previously. The *trend* in food poverty that emerged from the data was generally more positive. As Uvin (1994) summarized:

Until these data were published, it was commonly assumed that the proportion of hungry people in the world had declined slowly but consistently over the last decades, but that, as a result of population growth, the absolute number of the food poor had continued to grow. According to the new data, the absolute number of the food poor in the [developing] world has been declining since 1975, from 976 to 786 million persons in 1990. Food poverty has also been declining despite increasing numbers of nations which are not self-sufficient in food and the large number which are food short. Clearly, food shortage has not been an overriding determinant of food poverty.

Geographic overview by region
Nevertheless, trends in food poverty are more discouraging in regions where there is also food shortage. It would be surprising if this were not the case, since, if there is food shortage, at least some households must experience food poverty. Table 4.1 shows the trends in food poverty by region, using the same methodology for each time period.

The only region that has not experienced decline in the proportion of malnourished people – sub-Saharan Africa – is also a region where population growth was extremely high throughout the time period in question. The absolute numbers of malnourished people almost doubled between 1970 and 1990.

This is in contrast to South Asia, the other region for which dietary energy supply (DES) was insufficient in 1990 to provide everyone in the region with basic energy requirements (see table 3.2, p. 58). The absolute numbers in food poverty in South Asia have changed relatively little: 10 per cent fewer people in South Asia were in food poverty in 1990 than had been in 1970. Thus, South Asia has not experienced the declines in the absolute numbers in food poverty that most of the other regions have. This may be partly due to huge surges in basic grain production that have largely eliminated food shortage. But food poverty has not increased, even where shortage persists. This suggests there are many determinants of household access to food, other than its availability within the region.

Similar trends in Latin America support this more complex view: percentages in food poverty in Middle and South America from 1970 to 1990 declined a little, but the absolute numbers increased slightly. The trends occurred although the Latin American region as a whole is not food short. But structural-adjustment programmes implemented throughout the region during this era were one of the factors reducing access to food by poor households. Distribution-entitlement failures are most severe in Latin America and in the Near East and North Africa.

Overall, were China not included in the totals for developing regions, the trend in food poverty would not be positive. There were 156 million fewer chronically undernourished people in the developing world in 1990 than there had been in 1970; there were 217 million fewer in China. Sub-Saharan Africa is too sparsely populated to have the kind of impact on world totals that China or even India have. Although it is still accurate to summarize the trends in proportions of chronically undernourished as positive (sub-Saharan Africa was the only region to experience an increase, and this increase was only 2 per cent), the trends in absolute numbers of chronically undernourished are dominated by China and would not be positive if that nation were excluded.

Comparisons across population subgroups

In theory, the available data on food distribution across households could be used to determine *which* households are the most likely to suffer from food poverty. In practice, national-level data infrequently contain enough information about food distribution and/or information about the social and economic characteristics of the households to link this information. What we know about the types of households that are likely to suffer from food poverty comes primarily from small-scale surveys and community studies. It is very difficult to generalize from these about which households are hungry on a global or even regional basis, but they still provide important clues about the factors that increase hunger vulnerability.

Rural/urban differences

Important differences exist between rural and urban areas in the incidence of absolute poverty and food poverty, but the distinctions between these areas are not as clear as might be expected. Definitions of what constitutes an urban area are often left to the discretion of statistical offices within developing countries. Even employing fairly standard definitions, such as agglomerations of over 5,000 people, the physical size of the sustaining area is somewhat arbitrary. Some areas officially classified as urban have substantial proportions of their populations engaged in agriculture and may have more in common with rural villages than with central cities; this is particularly common in West Africa. Furthermore, circulation of families and individuals between rural and urban areas creates a group of people who cannot be unambiguously classified according to residence.

Although circular migrants' access to food has not been as intensively studied as other indicators of their well-being, such as infant mortality or adult literacy rates, those with urban exposure tend to be better off than their rural counterparts. This is one piece of the larger generalization that living in urban areas contributes to the health and well-being of populations. Health-care facilities are typically easier to reach for urban residents, who are also much more likely to have access to potable water, flush toilets, and refrigerators. Although access is unequal in urban areas, such amenities are entirely absent in many rural communities. Urban areas also (almost by definition) have better infrastructure for market and transport. The concentration of population also ensures more effective demand for food. All of these factors contribute to a picture of urban advantage for child survival, health, and access to food. For instance, when anthropometric measurements of young children are compared in developing countries, urban children frequently show stronger growth patterns than rural children (e.g. Bryceson 1989; Forster and Handelman 1985; Maher 1981). Additionally, larger proportions of the total (adult and child) population in rural areas have been found to be undernourished in many areas (e.g. Hossain 1987).

But food-consumption and expenditure surveys yield inconsistent results: some show that urbanities command better access to food (e.g. Uyanga 1979), while others document better access in rural areas (Walker and Ryan 1990). Throughout Latin America, more urbanized countries have greater food availability per capita, but data on the adequacy of energy intake between urban and rural dwellers still vary greatly (Uauy et al. 1984). Although food-consumption surveys often omit food consumed away from home – an occurrence that is somewhat likelier in urban areas – the failure of intake studies to show a consistent urban advantage highlights the possibility that conclusions based on growth outcomes may be heavily influenced by non-dietary factors such as sanitation, access to piped drinking water, and health services. Activity levels (and therefore caloric needs) may also be far lower for those engaged in urban occupations. In sum, the evidence of urban advantage in nutrition and its relationship to food poverty is mixed.

Within-rural variation
Not all rural households are equally dependent on agriculture for their livelihoods. Households that are involved in a diverse range of economic activities may be less vulnerable to entitlement failure than those with a single – or even a primary – source of entitlement. The following sections consider hunger vulnerability among rural groups with varying food strategies and entitlements.

LAND TENURE. Land ownership improves household food security in a number of ways. Owning any land gives households some measure of control over the means of production; owners can decide whether to consume or sell proceeds. It is especially important where markets are underdeveloped (Tschirley and Weber 1994). Owning land gives a guaranteed source of rural employment, although it does not guarantee that the source will be adequate to meet family food needs. Those who rely on cultivating their own land are less vulnerable to changes in rural wages but are still vulnerable to variations in rainfall, in costs of agricultural inputs, and in other forces affecting their productivity.

One of the most consistent findings from the literature on land tenure and nutritional status is that rural households that own any land are better off than those that do not (Alderman and von Braun 1984; Forster and Handelman 1985; Lipton and Longhurst 1989; Melville 1988; Victora et al. 1986; Walker and Ryan 1990). Land ownership serves as a proxy for household wealth, and therefore its relationship with favourable nutritional status does prove that land enhances food security. However, there is also a considerable body of evidence indicating that landed households are less vulnerable to hunger, in cases of production shortfalls, than are rural labourers (Sen 1981a).

However, absolute size of holding is obviously important. What absolute size is required for food security will depend on local ecological, political, and economic conditions; on household needs; and on other sources of income. In areas where landholding has become fragmented, typical holdings are likely to be inadequate. A study of six poor villages in Bangladesh concluded that at least half an acre was needed to provide basic needs for an average family, but very few families had access to that much land (Hossain 1987). Similarly, Griffin (1976) estimated that 90 per cent of the landholdings in Guatemala were too small for subsistence. This pattern is typical in Latin America, where much land is held as large estates (Sheahan 1987).

A number of studies have shown that households that own more land have lower rates of child malnutrition (DeWalt et al. 1987; Fleuret and Fleuret 1980; Gopalan 1987; Grewal et al. 1973; Victora and Vaughan 1985), yet it is difficult to conclude from this evidence that larger holdings *increase* household food security because plot size may simply be a proxy for wealth, and the definitions of small and large holdings employed vary widely in these studies. Furthermore, other studies show holding size to be uncorrelated with nutritional status (see reviews in Melville 1988 and Victora et al. 1986), and childhood malnutrition can occur independently of household food poverty. Owning more land is most likely to protect against food poverty where holdings are large enough to accommodate a range of production strategies and therefore decrease risk.

Rural households that do not own enough land to meet their needs may gain access to additional land as hired labour or through tenant or sharecropping arrangements. The type of access to unowned land influences household food security, and sharecroppers and tenants both generally have more control over food than hired labourers, who are less likely to have customary patronage protection to fall back on in case of crop failure (Sen 1981b). Secure tenant farmers in India own their own draught animals (Walker and Ryan 1990) and have access to other resources. Those who are better off to start with are able to benefit more from arrangements that give them access to land that they do not own. However, those engaged in wage labour may suffer fewer income fluctuations because they are also likely to be engaged in non-agricultural employment (Walker and Ryan 1990). In addition, sharecropping arrangements are shrinking as landowners adopt modern agricultural inputs (Alavi 1973).

Overall, land ownership can be expected to matter most where access to land is most heavily governed by ownership. This rather obvious conclusion is sometimes overlooked in the generalizations drawn from studies of landholding in various settings. De Waal (1989) showed that, in the Sudan, pastoralists who had access to a great deal of land were better protected in times of drought than their more wealthy agriculturist neighbours. They were able to change herd compositions and they knew more about wild foods than farmers did. Landlessness, and insecure access to land, threaten food security most in rural communities in which productive assets are privately controlled. Although restricted access to land is still far less of a problem in Africa than in other developing areas, landlessness is growing in Africa as a result of privatization (Jazairy et al. 1992), and other forces are increasing landlessness in the Near East and Latin America.

Additionally, the focus on land tenure should not obscure the importance of livestock in family subsistence strategies. Not all farm families own livestock, and many landless households nevertheless own draught animals, milch animals, or smaller livestock. These can be another store of wealth and also an important source of food. During the 1983 drought in Zimbabwe, households that owned live-stock were one-third less likely to require food aid than households *of the same income level* that did not (Gittinger et al. 1990). Being able to sell animals in times of severe drought can make a critical difference for households whose income would be otherwise inade-quate to secure entitlement to food. Although selling livestock has the potential to increase vulnerability to hunger in the future, in some settings buyers protect animals by removing them from regions too dry to support them and then reselling them back into these regions later (Rahmato 1988).

CASH-CROPPING. Cash-cropping has long been a suspected contributor to undernutrition. Cash crops are alleged to have the following effects:
1. They cause greater environmental degradation than food crops (ACC/SCN 1989; Schofield 1975; Van Esterik 1984).

2. They increase the maldistribution of land (George 1977; Melville 1988; Taussig 1978).
3. They take better lands away from crops (Güsten 1968; Wright T. C. 1985).
4. They divert labour from food production (Forster and Handelman 1985; Hamilton et al. 1984; Schofield 1979) and preparation (Schofield 1975).
5. They increase the energy that must be expended to obtain the same nutrients (Fleuret and Fleuret 1980).
6. They render cash-crop producers vulnerable to world market prices (Van Esterik 1984).
7. They increase debt through elevated use of credit (Van Esterik 1984).
8. They divert income from food (Brandtzaeg 1982; Rogers and Youssef 1988; Schofield 1979).
9. They increase use of foods with low nutrient value (Suárez et al. 1987).
10. They lead to irregular intakes because of irregular income (Fleuret and Fleuret 1980; Kaiser and Dewey 1991; Trenchard 1987; von Braun et al. 1994).
11. They decrease dietary diversity (Dewey 1985; Schofield 1979; Taussig 1978).

The first three of these reasons refer more to global than household impacts. The use of better lands for marketed crops reduces global food security only if the marketed crops are products such as sisal and tobacco rather than food. But even factors that primarily affect global production and productive potential influence food distribution across households.

Commercial agriculture has the potential to increase household vulnerability to hunger, because access to food then depends on markets and prices rather than production. But extensive literature reviews have not concluded that cash-cropping is uniformly bad for nutrition (Mebrahtu et al. 1995), and the Latin American evidence points to a mix of subsistence and cash-cropping as the best nutritional strategy (Messer 1984). Fairly compelling reasons why cash-cropping could improve nutritional status include the provision of producers with revenue to improve agricultural productivity and the increase in employment opportunities for the rural landless.

Mixed findings on the effects of cash-cropping on household food security are partly explained by the substantial variation in its effects according to local conditions. Bryceson (1989) argued that cash-cropping tends to be somewhat less risky in Africa because better land availability allows cash-croppers to return to subsistence cultivation when market terms of trade deteriorate. Similarly, cash-cropping is less risky where conditions allow farmers to combine food and cash crops, as where coffee and bananas are intercropped (Bryceson 1989). As in Latin America, cash-cropping families that have the most secure nutritional status are those that have diversified their production, particularly those who also grow food for their own consumption (FAO 1986; Melville 1988).

But crop diversification, particularly in Africa, may be constrained by labour availability. Where male labour is diverted into cash-crop production, women are left with the responsibilities of food production, food preparation, and child care. Nutrition suffers where any of these three responsibilities is neglected or compromised. Household access to food may also decline where women's heavier participation in subsistence agriculture limits the time they have available for remunerated activities. In much of sub-Saharan Africa, women are responsible for providing food for their families and men's earnings are not spent on food (Bryson 1981; Desai 1992; Guyer 1984; Lloyd and Brandon 1991; Seidman 1984). A shift to cash-cropping may mean that increased income comes at the expense of increased food expenditure, because the proceeds from cash crops are controlled by men (Bukh 1979; FAO 1987; Trenchard 1987).

Although these factors explain some of the variable findings on the impact of cash-cropping on nutritional status, some of the ambiguity arises from focusing on the nutritional outcomes for different groups. The effects of cash-cropping on those involved in the process differ greatly from those on others in the community.

Where cash crops affect food supply, their impact depends on how diets resulting from purchasing food with the revenues from cash crops compare with diets based on production. Increased production, even of food crops that are then sold for cash, can threaten food supply and nutrition, as where indigenous cultivators of highland Ecuador trade legumes for flour and lard. In many cases, agricultural commodities produced for the market are not consumed locally (Schofield 1979); local diets have been shown to be increasingly dependent on staple grains and therefore lacking in micronutrients (Abdullah 1988). But, in some areas, commercial production is associated with more diverse local diets (e.g. Glover 1994) that are protective against micronutrient deficiencies. Commercialization that brings with it increased investment in agricultural research and development, extension, and improved marketing increase production incentives and total food supply and potentially reduce food poverty indirectly by reducing food shortage.

Nevertheless, cash-cropping has greater potential to influence food poverty through food prices, labour prices, and land distribution. Landowning households that produce a diverse set of crops for the market are less vulnerable to fluctuating market prices and failures of particular crops. Continuing subsistence production protects cash-cropping households with a source of entitlement to food besides income. Cash-cropping tends to be associated with good nutritional outcomes in these households.

The effects of cash-cropping on non-participating households are more complicated. Rural households with smallholdings may continue to specialize in subsistence production because they cannot afford the risk or the investment necessary to compete with larger-scale commercial farmers. If productivity in the rest of the agricultural sector drives prices down, these households will receive less income from whatever surplus they sell. This increases their costs for food purchases and the amounts they need to sell in order to meet their other cash needs, including taxes. Wealthier households – especially those with larger landholdings – are the most likely to benefit from subsidies and credit programmes. Cash-cropping tends to augment the nutritional status of participating households, in part because those who participate are already in the best positions to diversify production and therefore to minimize the inherent risks.

The effects of cash-cropping on *landless* households are mixed. Cash-cropping often increases the demand for agricultural labour and thereby increases the incomes of rural landless labourers, but the availability and financial returns from expanding wage work depends on the labour supply competing for the new jobs. Where smallholders and outsiders enter in search of employment, cash-cropping schemes can lower wages.

Where cash-cropping drives down food prices, urban dwellers can be expected to enjoy improved food security, if earnings remain stable. Where cash-cropping absorbs labour and does not provide an impetus for rural-to-urban migration, the urban poor can benefit from less competition for jobs. But where, instead, capital-intensive cash-cropping displaces rural wage labour, sending more to the city in search of work, commercialization reduces wages and food security for the urban poor.

Measurements of the impacts of large-scale commercial changes in agriculture on particular population groups tend to be purely academic. Von Braun (1994) has argued that subsistence agriculture is ceasing to be a viable alternative for individual producers and for the global economy. Although analysts tend to assess whether farmers would have been better off remaining in subsistence production, the more important policy question is how to protect particular groups during the transition. Social safety nets are very important in protecting groups such as tenants and smallholders, who lose customary sources of entitlement during large-scale commercial transformations and may not yet have acquired new modes of livelihood.

SEASONALITY. A pattern of fluctuating rural intakes across agricultural seasons has been documented in a wide variety of countries and has been well known for decades (Chambers et al. 1981; Schofield 1974). The basic cause for this pattern is simply lower food availability during "hungry" seasons before harvesting reverses the situation into one of plenty. Even if food intake were constant across seasons, there would still be lower intake relative to need during harvesting because energy expenditure is high during peak agricultural work times.

Although seasonality in food intake is directly related to seasonality in agriculture, there are still important questions with respect to the role of seasonality in influencing food poverty. Are there some rural households that have less-dramatic fluctuations in intake? Are there households that, despite fluctuations, still have adequate intake at every point in the year? The answers to these questions are not known on a global scale, but there is some indication that even wealthy landholders do not have consistent intakes across agricultural seasons (Abdullah 1988; Walker and Ryan 1990). Own production does not safeguard against seasonal hunger as well as it does against more chronic hunger.

Entitlement to food on a year-round basis depends on total production and access to adequate storage facilities, and on effective demand to buy extra food. Markets are a cost-effective solution to seasonal food availability where there is sufficient purchasing power. Money stores better than food, but access to markets in remote rural areas is limited by distance and undeveloped infrastructure; food prices can rise quickly during hungry seasons when demand for purchased food is high. As indicated above, even where markets and commercialized production provide greater quantities of cheaper staple foods, they do not necessarily offer optimal year-round nutrition. Greater consumption of rice throughout the year can be accompanied by greater seasonal vitamin and mineral deprivation; and the very poor may still find they suffer chronic, as opposed to seasonal, hunger.

Within-urban variation
Urban nutritional variation tends to be related to employment, although health and dietary choices are other factors. Jobs in the formal sector tend to pay higher wages than productive activities in the informal economy. Formal-sector jobs also provide more stable income, since wages do not fluctuate in the same way as self-employment earnings. But many who migrate to urban areas fail to find formal-sector employment; they return to the countryside, or continue to try to find a job while being supported by their families, or engage in informal activities, or employ some combination of these strategies.

When the wage and income disparities between rural and urban areas are minimal, the incentives to move and remain underemployed in urban areas diminishes, but urban underemployment and demand for government services remain a persistent problem in most countries in the developing world. Rural development is the most promising method to limit migration and urban blight, since it changes the economic opportunity structure and improves access to social services, rather than trying to constrain rational responses to existing structures. But even countries facing urban crowding have failed to invest the high direct costs of developing rural infrastructure and jobs, in part for lack of funds and in part out of a desire to maintain low urban wages to promote industry. Industrialists provide a far stronger power base for politicians than do the rural poor. Although long-run strategies for promoting integrated national development are desirable for a number of reasons, the poor and growing urban class that is vulnerable to hunger also demands short-run attention. The urban lower class is not limited to those living in squatter settlements or those who have recently migrated to urban areas; however, both because these two groups are easily defined and because there are strong reasons for believing that they might be disadvantaged, their hunger status has been fairly widely studied.

SQUATTER SETTLEMENTS. Consumption surveys have shown, not surprisingly, that urban squatters consume less energy and have a greater prevalence of vitamin deficiencies than any other urban class (Gopalan 1987; Rao 1987). In the Philippines, the average family wage among urban squatters covered only 87 per cent of the cost of a minimum basic diet (Eviota 1986).

Squatters living in large cities sometimes have an advantage, in that more government subsidies are available to them (Alderman and von Braun 1984). However, benefits diminish with distance: those furthest from the urban centre tend to have the highest rates of malnutrition (Wright E. W. 1985). The perpetuation of social inequality that leads to food poverty is difficult to overcome in situations like this. Those living on the urban fringes are usually less economically productive, as they spend more of their time reaching markets and jobs. In addition, squatters may be vulnerable to eviction, or to cut-off of water, electricity, or other services. Generally substandard housing, lack of sanitation, and denial of entitlements to social welfare programmes including free or low-cost health services and access to subsidized food – all these conditions perpetuate social inequality and hunger.

MIGRANTS. Nutritional outcomes may vary greatly between recent and established migrants; they may vary greatly between circular and permanent migrants; and they may vary greatly between visitors and those intending to stay. Migrants (urban dwellers who were not urban born) as a group appear to be better off than those living in squatter settlements, even though some migrants may be urban squatters. Migration is rarely undertaken by individuals in isolation. Many stay and eat with urban contacts while they are looking for employment (Skeldon 1990). These urban relations also help them to find jobs, sometimes locating employment for them even before they leave their rural homes (Fawcett et al. 1984). Money and/or food sent to urban migrants from rural relatives also helps support the migrant's search for a formal-sector job (Fuller et al. 1990). Because migration often takes significant resources to launch, migrants also sometimes start off at an economic advantage relative to the urban poor: they may represent the rural wealthy rather than the rural or urban poor. In sum, as a group they are not at as high a risk for food insecurity as many more-established, but poor, urban dwellers. Definitional problems, coupled with the fact that migrant intentions are not always clear (and not always followed through on when clear), make studying food intake among migrants particularly problematic.

119

Case study: The importance of non-market entitlements

Although it is entirely predictable that households with fewer resources and productive assets are more likely to be food poor, it is far less predictable which of the millions of impoverished households in the developing world will be unable to provide food for all of their members under normal circumstances, or which are best equipped to survive crisis conditions. In food-insecure environments, the ability of households to avoid food poverty depends critically on their ability to minimize risk. This entails a diversification of entitlement strategies, but the hunger literature has focused far more on production-based, market-based, and government-provided entitlements than it has on non-market exchanges, which are part of the "moral economy." Some have argued that non-market access to food is becoming a less-important survival strategy as production systems become more cash oriented and integrated into national economies; Collier (1990) showed that cash transactions were replacing labour and food exchange in a highland Mexican community. But others find that non-market sources of entitlement are still crucial for many households, and the ability to obtain food through non-market channels helps to explain why, at the same income level, some households are food poor while others are not.

Adams' detailed study of Bambara households in central Mali (Adams 1993) illustrates just how essential social and affective ties are in safeguarding vulnerable households against hunger. The poorest households were more likely to give food away under normal circumstances. They used their gifts to create ties to more prosperous households which, in turn, sustained them with food when production was limited by scant rains. Non-market exchanges among the Bambara extended beyond the village, through marriage ties that created additional obligations to share food. These inter-village linkages were particularly important during times of crisis: when food shortage weakened intra-village lineage networks through household fission and migration, cereals provided by in-laws became crucial for subsistence (Adams 1993).

Affective ties between farmers and traders also proved to be important during times of food shortage: loyal clients of local traders were extended uncustomary credit and even employment opportunities (Adams 1993).

In sum, non-market entitlements to food were secured in three main ways by Bambara households: these were from cereal gifts, exchange of labour for cereal, and use of non-market credit (Adams 1993). Together, these strategies provided food for almost a quarter of the food-short days during the weak 1988/89 agricultural year. For households on the receiving end, non-market transactions met about half of their food needs, so non-market exchange was far from being a trivial part of household subsistence strategies. Although Adams showed that some Bambara households did not participate actively in non-market labour and food exchange because they devoted more of their resources to cash-cropping (a pattern that has also been documented elsewhere [Collier 1990]), the modern exchange economy has not completely eroded more traditional patterns of exchange.

Relationships that appear to be market based but are also governed by strong affective and moral ties during times of food scarcity have parallels in other African (Valentine 1993) and non-African (Payne et al. 1994) countries. The importance of non-market transfers in Botswana is particularly noteworthy because public assistance (made possible largely through diamond wealth) has been noted as a crucial part of drought relief. Even with public assistance widely available, Valentine (1993) showed that private non-market transfers were an important factor in maintaining the same (relatively low) level of income inequality across drought and non-drought years.

Policy recommendations to reduce food poverty

Trends in world food poverty are encouraging: despite rapid population growth, there are fewer households now that cannot afford to feed all of their members than in recent decades. From what we know about who is hungry, we can also identify ways to reduce food poverty further among the approximately 786 million that are still food poor, for whom the positive trend so far makes little difference.

More effective monitoring efforts

Famine early warning systems include highly technological components, such as atmospheric monitoring, but they are based on the knowledge that food scarcity changes the way households meet their food needs. Under the most austere conditions, coping strategies include divesting wealth and finally selling off productive assets in order to meet short-run food needs. Information about sale of such assets as jewellery and livestock is gathered to identify areas where hunger is very likely to occur.

These monitoring efforts are not particularly costly, given how much more effectively interventions can be targeted with better knowledge of which populations are affected. Nevertheless, the cost of monitoring is much higher than it needs to be, because some areas are covered by two or more monitoring programmes. Duplication wastes resources that could be used for combating hunger and sometimes also delays relief action. During the 1991/92 Southern African drought, estimates of food needs were prepared by local monitoring agencies, but distribution of relief supplies did not begin until international agencies also had conducted their own monitoring efforts (Callihan et al. 1994). Coordination of efforts would save both money and time.

Longer time-frames for structural adjustment

The magnitude of the effect of structural-adjustment programmes on income distribution in developing countries was not fully appreciated when the first programmes were implemented. The Social Dimensions of Adjustment project, and other poverty-alleviation programmes that now typically accompany structural adjustment, have taken important steps toward reducing the human suffering that accompanies adjustment. However, for the most part these poverty-alleviation elements are simply add-ons rather than being integral to the adjustment plans that still reduce employment and access to subsidized food (Jolly 1988).

For adjusting countries to comply with conditions of structural adjustment without leaving large segments of their populations more vulnerable to hunger, poverty-alleviation programmes should be coordinated with the broader adjustment goals. This will usually mean that the adjustment process needs to proceed more slowly than currently typical timetables allow (Jolly 1988). If the goal of structural adjustment is to alter the fundamental production and consumption structures so that the economy will function in a sustainable way, the longer time-frames will make success more likely; if the primary goal of structural adjustment is, in fact, debt repayment, longer programmes have little political chance of succeeding.

More employment programmes

Creating employment through public works projects or promotion of more labour-intensive technologies in the private sector enhances household command over food through wage-based entitlements. Public employment programmes supplement earning opportunities during times of structural transition and are especially important under conditions of extreme food and employment scarcity, including post-war reconstruction (Callihan et al. 1994). After conflict has ceased, household wherewithal to secure food can be strengthened by operating programmes that replace lost sources of entitlement. Food-for-work or cash-for-work programmes can also be used to rebuild food-distribution infrastructure damaged by violent conflict.

More emphasis on rural development

A primary cause of urban poverty is rural poverty. Poor employment options in the rural sector contribute to migration, even where urban areas are already overcrowded. Urban jobs, when available, tend to be better remunerated than rural jobs, and even the underemployed tend to fare better in urban areas because they have better access to government food-distribution programmes, public health-care facilities, and education. More equitable distribution of public programmes would reduce incentives for rural-to-urban migration and contribute to sustaining a diversified set of food entitlements for rural households. Better health care in rural areas would also decrease household hunger by increasing worker productivity and individual ability to utilize food efficiently. Public investment to generate greater employment and private-sector industry in rural areas would benefit households that still engage in subsistence agriculture but that cannot meet all of their need in that way (Meier 1989).

Increasing employment and income in the agricultural sector must also be a priority. Government low-cost-food pricing and marketing policies that limit incentives for food production and rural incomes should be modified. National food availability and the livelihoods of agriculturists could be simultaneously improved if prices for food crops were not held artificially low. Furthermore, government programmes that emphasize basic food production as well as export promotion could eliminate cascading effects of national-level food shortages on food poverty.

Improved rural access to credit
Skewed income distribution in rural areas often is reinforced by participation in the market economy. Those who start out best situated multiply their productivity and wealth by early adoption of modern

agricultural inputs. Small landholders without investment capital or margin for risk are left far behind. Government export promotion favours those growing cash crops and helps to institutionalize a bimodal pattern of agricultural development where only one segment is benefiting from change.

Rural financial institutions and credit programmes targeted at poorer farmers can help interrupt growing social inequality and vulnerability to hunger by making credit available to those unable to secure it on normal commercial terms. Even where smallholders are not favoured in the distribution of credit, better rural finance and credit infrastructure could help smooth seasonal fluctuations in income and accompanying seasonal patterns of hunger. Secure financial institutions also could increase the reliability of migrant remittances, since transferring income back to rural areas would be less risky. All are programmes that might constrain household poverty, and thereby give all individuals in poor households a greater pie from which to bargain their fair share.

Summary and conclusions

This chapter has shown that there are more food-poor households in food-short regions but that there are also substantial numbers of food-poor households in food-adequate regions. Rural households are more likely to be food poor than urban ones. Within rural areas, the main factors associated with food poverty are as follows: undiversified production; low food prices for rural produce coupled with high prices for other commodities; excessive taxation; low revenues for cash crops without compensating low food prices; lack of transport and market opportunities; lack of control over resource endowments such as land; low exchange entitlements (wages); and lack of alternative employment opportunities and sources of income. Within urban areas, food poverty is related to underemployment and poor remuneration, but it also results in part from substandard housing, unhygienic living conditions, and lack of access to health care.

Short-term relief projects can temporarily improve submarginal household incomes. Longer-term adjustment programmes are designed to strengthen private-sector investment and make government programmes more cost-effective. But, in the short term, transition economies tend to have more food-poor households that need special social programmes to avoid food poverty.

Food-poor households often compromise their longer-run security in order to survive the short run. They also face decisions about whether to put some members at a relative disadvantage in order to protect the health and earning capacity of others. The following chapter evaluates evidence for systematic discrimination in the allocation of food to individuals within households; it gives special attention to differences between crisis situations and normal conditions, and also compares the distribution patterns within food-poor households with those in food-adequate ones.

Works cited

Abdullah, Mohammad. 1988. "Modernization of Agriculture and Seasonality of Food Intake." *Nutrition Reports International* 37, No. 6: 1147–1159.

ACC/SCN. 1989. "Does Cash Cropping Affect Nutrition?" *SCN News* No. 3: 2–10.

———. 1992. *Second Report on the World Nutrition Situation; Volume I Global and Regional Results*. Geneva: Administrative Committee on Coordination, Subcommittee on Nutrition.

Adams, Alayne. 1993. "Food Insecurity in Mali: Exploring the Role of the Moral Economy." *IDS Bulletin* 24, No. 4: 41–51.

Alavi, Hamza. 1973. "Elite Farmer Strategy and Regional Disparities in the Agricultural Development of Pakistan." *Economic and Political Weekly* VIII, No. 13: A-31–A-39.

Alderman, Harold, and Joachim von Braun. 1984. "The Effects of the Egyptian Food Ration and Subsidy System on Income Distribution and Consumption." *IFPRI Research Report*, No. 45.

Brandtzaeg, Brita. 1982. "The Role and Status of Women and Post-Harvest Food Conservation." *Food and Nutrition Bulletin* 4: 33–40.

Bryceson, Deborah Fahy. 1989. "Nutrition and the Commoditization of Food in Sub-Saharan Africa." *Social Science and Medicine* 28, No. 5: 425–440.

Bryson, Judy C. 1981. "Women and Agriculture in Sub-Saharan Africa: Implications for Development (an Exploratory Study)." *Journal of Development Studies* 17, No. 3: 29–46.

Bukh, Jette. 1979. *The Village Woman in Ghana*. Copenhagen: Centre for Development Research.

Callihan, David M., John H. Eriksen, and Allison Butler Herrick. 1994. *Famine Averted: The United States Government Response to the 1991/92 Southern Africa Drought*. Management Systems International, Evaluation Synthesis Report Prepared for USAID/Bureau for Humanitarian Response. Washington, D.C.: Management Systems International.

Chambers, Robert, Richard Longhurst, and Arnold Pacey, eds. 1981. *Seasonal Dimensions to Rural Poverty*. London: F. Pinter and Totowa, N.J.: Allenheld, Osmun.

Chen, Martha Alter. 1991. *Coping with Seasonality and Drought*. New Delhi: Sage.

Collier, George A. 1990. *Seeking Food and Seeking Money: Changing Productive Relations in a Highland Mexican Community*. United Nations Research Institute for Social Development, Discussion Paper 11. Geneva: UNRISD.

de Waal, Alexander. 1989. *Famine That Kills: Darfur, Sudan, 1984–1985*. Oxford: Clarendon Press, and New York: Oxford University Press.

Desai, Sonalde. 1992. "Children at Risk: The Role of Family Structure in Latin America and West Africa." *Population and Development Review* 18, No. 4: 689–717.

DeWalt, Billie R., Kathleen M. DeWalt, José Carlos Escudero, and David Barkin. 1987. "Agrarian Reform and Small-Farmer Welfare: Evidence from Four Mexican Communities." *Food and Nutrition Bulletin* 9, No. 3: 46–52.

Dewey, Kathryn G. 1985. "Nutritional Consequences of the Transformation from Subsistence to Commercial Agriculture in Tabasco, Mexico." In: Dorothy J. Cattle and Karl H. Schwerin, eds. *Food Energy in Tropical Ecosystems*. New York: Gordon and Breach, pp. 105–144.

Drèze, Jean, and Amartya Sen. 1990. "Introduction." In: Jean Drèze and Amartya Sen, eds. *The Political Economy of Hunger*, Volume I. Oxford: Clarendon Press, pp. 1–33.

Eviota, Elizabeth U. 1986. "The Articulation of Gender and Class in the Philippines." In: Eleanor Leacock, Helen I. Safa, and contributors, eds. *Women's Work: Development and the Division of Labor by Gender*. South Hadley, Massachusetts: Bergin & Garvey, pp. 194–206.

FAO. 1986. *Kenya*. Food and Agriculture Organization of the United Nations, ESNA – Nutrition Country Profile. Rome: FAO.

———. 1987. "Women in African Food Production and Security." In: J. Price Gittinger, Joanne Leslie, and Caroline Hoisington, eds. *Food Policy: Integrating Supply, Distribution, and Consumption*. Baltimore: Johns Hopkins University Press, pp. 133–140.

Fawcett, James T., Siew-Ean Koo, and Peter C. Smith, eds. 1984. *Women in the Cities of Asia: Migration and Urban Adaptation*. Boulder, Colorado: Westview Press.

Findley, Sally E. 1994. "Does Drought Increase Migration: A Study of Rural Mali during the 1983–85 Drought." *International Migration Review* 28 (Fall): 539–553.

Fleuret, Patrick, and Anne Fleuret. 1980. "Nutrition, Consumption, and Agricultural Change." *Human Organization* 39, No. 3: 250–260.

Forster, Nancy, and Howard Handelman. 1985. "Food Production and Distribution in Cuba: The Impact of the Revolution." In: John C. Super and Thomas C. Wright, eds. *Food, Politics, and Society in Latin America*. Lincoln: University of Nebraska Press, pp. 65–105.

Fuller, Theodore D., P. Kamnuansilpa, and Paul Lightfoot. 1990. "Urban Ties of Rural Thais." *International Migration Review* 24, (Fall): 534–562.

George, Susan. 1977. *How the Other Half Dies: The Real Reasons for World Hunger*. Montclair, New Jersey: Allanheld, Osmun.

Gittinger, J. Price, Sidney Chernick, Nadine R. Horenstein, and Katrine Saito. 1990. "Household Food Security and the Role of Women." *World Bank Discussion Papers*, No. 96. Washington, D.C.: World Bank.

Glover, David. 1994. "Contract Farming and Commercialization of Agriculture in Developing Countries." In: Joachim von Braun and Eileen Kennedy, eds. *Agricultural Commercialization, Economic Development, and Nutrition*. Baltimore: Johns Hopkins University Press, pp. 166–175.

Goldscheider, Calvin, ed. 1983. *Urban Migrants in Developing Nations: Patterns and Problems of Adjustment*. Brown University Studies in Population and Development. Boulder, Colorado: Westview Press.

Gopalan, C. 1987. "Heights of Populations – an Index of Their Nutrition and Socio-economic Development." *NFI Bulletin: Bulletin of the Nutrition Foundation of India* 8, No. 3: 1–5.

Grewal, Tina, Tara Gopaldes, and V. J. Gadre. 1973. "Etiology of Malnutrition in Rural Indian Preschool Children (Madhya Pradesh)." *Environmental Child Health* 19: 265–270.

Griffin, Keith. 1976. *Land Concentration and Rural Poverty*. London: Macmillan.

Güsten, Rolf. 1968. *Studies in the Staple Food Economy of Western Nigeria*. Vol. 30. Afrika-Studien, series ed. Ifo-Institut für Wirtschafts-forschung. Munich: Welt-forum Verlag.

Guyer, Jane I. 1984. *Family and Farm in Southern Cameroon*. Vol. 15. African Research Studies, Boston: African Studies Center, Boston University.

Hamilton, Sahni, Barry Popkin, and Deborah Spicer. 1984. *Women and Nutrition in Third World Countries*. Praeger Special Studies. New York: Bergin & Garvey.

Hossain, Mosharaff. 1987. *The Assault that Failed: A Profile of Absolute Poverty in Six Villages of Bangladesh*. Geneva: United Nations Research Institute for Social Development.

Jazairy, Idriss, Mohiuddin Alamgir, and Theresa Panuccio. 1992. *The State of World Rural Poverty: An Inquiry into Its Causes and Consequences*. New York: New York University Press.

Jolly, Richard. 1988. "Poverty and Adjustment in the 1990s." In: John P. Lewis, ed. *Strengthening the Poor: What Have We Learned?* New Brunswick: Transaction Books, pp. 163–175.

Kaiser, L. L., and K. G. Dewey. 1991. "Household Economic Strategies and Food Expenditure Patterns in Rural Mexico: Impact on Nutritional Status of Preschool Children." *Ecology of Food and Nutrition* 25: 147–168.

Kates, Robert W. 1996. "Ending Hunger: 1999 and Beyond." In: Ellen Messer and Peter Uvin, eds. *The Hunger Report: 1995*. Amsterdam: Gordon and Breach, pp. 229–245.

Lipton, Michael, and Richard Longhurst. 1989. *New Seeds and Poor People*. Baltimore: Johns Hopkins University Press.

Lloyd, Cynthia B., and Anastasia Brandon. 1991. *Women's Role in Maintaining Households: Poverty and Gender Inequality in Ghana*. Population Council, Research Division Working Papers No. 25. New York: Population Council.

Macedo, Roberto. 1988. "Brazilian Children and the Economic Crisis: The Evidence from the State of Saõ Paulo." In: Giovanni Andrea Cornia, Richard Jolly, and Frances Stewart, eds. *Adjustment with a Human Face: Volume II, Country Case Studies*. Oxford: Clarendon Press, pp. 28–56.

Maher, Vanessa. 1981. "Work, Consumption and Authority with the Household." In: Kate Young, Carol Wolkowitz, and Roslyn McCullagh, eds. *Of Marriage and the Market: Women's Subordination in International Perspective*. London: CSE Books, pp. 69–87.

Mebrahtu, Saba, David Pelletier, and Per Pinstrup-Andersen. 1995. "Agriculture and Nutrition." In: Per Pinstrup-Andersen, David Pelletier, and Harold Alder-man, eds. *Child Growth and Nutrition in Developing Countries*. Ithaca: Cornell University Press, pp. 220–242.

Meier, Gerald M., ed. 1989. *Leading Issues in Economic Development*. Fifth Edition. New York: Oxford University Press.

Melville, Bendley F. 1988. "Are Land Availability and Cropping Pattern Critical Factors in Determining Nutritional Status?" *Food and Nutrition Bulletin* 10, No. 2: 44–48.

Messer, Ellen. 1984. "Anthropological Perspectives on Diet." *Annual Review of Anthropology* 13: 205–250.

Payne, Philip, Michael Lipton, Richard Longhurst, James North, and Steven Treagust. 1994. *How Third World Rural Households Adapt to Dietary Energy Stress: The Evidence and the Issues*. Vol. 2. IFPRI Food Policy Reviews. Washington, D.C.: International Food Policy Research Institute.

Quinn, Victoria, Mark Cohen, John Mason, and B. N. Kgosidintsi. 1988. "Crisis-Proofing the Economy: The Response of Botswana to Economic Recession and Drought." In: Giovanni Andrea Cornia, Richard Jolly, and Frances Stewart, eds. *Adjustment with a Human Face: Volume II, Country Case Studies*. Oxford: Clarendon Press, pp. 3–27.

Rahmato, Dessalegn. 1988. "Peasant Survival Strategies in Ethiopia." *Disasters* 12, No. 4: 326–344.

Rao, Kamala S. Jaya. 1987. "Urban Nutrition in India – II." In: C. Gopalan, ed. *Combating Undernutrition: Basic Issues and Practical Approaches*. Hyderabad: Nutrition Foundation of India, pp. 314–320.

Ravallion, Martin. 1987. *Markets and Famines*. Oxford: Clarendon Press.

Rogers, Beatrice Lorge. 1995. "Feeding Programs and Food-Related Income Transfers." In: Per Pinstrup-Andersen, David Pelletier, and Harold Alderman, eds. *Child Growth and Nutrition in Developing Countries*. Ithaca: Cornell University Press, pp. 199–219.

———, and Nadia Youssef. 1988. "The Importance of Women's Involvement in Economic Activities in the Improvement of Child Nutrition and Health." *Food and Nutrition Bulletin* 10, No. 3: 33–41.

Schofield, S. 1974. "Seasonal Factors Affecting Nutrition in Different Age Groups and Especially Pre-School Children." *Journal of Development Studies* I: 22–40.

———. 1975. *Village Nutrition Studies: An Annotated Bibliography*. Brighton, UK: Institute of Development Studies at the University of Sussex.

———. 1979. *Development and the Problems of Village Nutrition*. Montclair, New Jersey: Allanheld, Osmun.

Seaman, John. 1993. "Famine Mortality in Africa." *IDS Bulletin* 24, No. 4: 27–32.

Seidman, Gay W. 1984. "Women in Zimbabwe: Postindependence Struggles." *Feminist Studies* 10, No. 3: 419–440.

Sen, Amartya K. 1981a. "Ingredients of Famine Analysis: Availability and Entitlements." *Quarterly Journal of Economics* XCVI, No. 3: 433–464.

———. 1981b. *Poverty and Famines: An Essay on Entitlement and Deprivation*. Oxford: Clarendon Press.

Serageldin, Ismail. 1990. "The Human Dimension of Structural Adjustment Programmes: The World Bank's Perspective." In: Adebayo Adedeji, Sadig Rasheed, and Melody Morrison, eds. *The Human Dimension of Africa's Persistent Economic Crisis*. London: Hans Zell, pp. 237–260.

Sheahan, John. 1987. *Patterns of Development in Latin America*. Princeton, New Jersey: Princeton University Press.

Skeldon, Ronald. 1990. *Population Mobility in Developing Countries*. New York: Belhaven Press.

Suárez, B., D. Barkin, B. DeWalt, M. Hernández, and R. Rosales. 1987. "The Nutritional Impact of Rural Modernization: Strategies for Smallholder Survival in Mexico." *Food and Nutrition Bulletin* 9, No. 3: 30–35.

Taussig, Michael. 1978. "Peasant Economies and the Development of Capitalist Agriculture in the Cauca Valley, Colombia." *Latin American Perspectives* 5, No. 3: 62–90.

Trenchard, Esther. 1987. "Rural Women's Work in Sub-Saharan Africa and the Implications for Nutrition." In: Janet Henshall Momsen and Janet G. Townsend, eds. *Geography of Gender in the Third World*. Hutchinson: State University of New York Press, pp. 153–172.

Tschirley, David L., and Michael T. Weber. 1994. "Food Security Strategies Under Extremely Adverse Conditions: The Determinants of Household Income and Consumption in Rural Mozambique." *World Development* 22, No. 2: 159–173.

Uauy, Ricardo, Rolando Chateauneuf, and Sergio Valiente. 1984. "Food and Nutrition Problems in Urbanized Latin America: Misdirected Development." In: Philip L. White and Nancy Selvey, eds. *Malnutrition: Determinants and Consequences*. Proceedings of the Western Hemisphere Nutrition Congress VII. New York: Alan R. Liss, pp. 29–43.

Uvin, Peter. 1994. "The State of World Hunger." *Nutrition Reviews* 52, No. 5: 151–161.

Uyanga, Joseph. 1979. "Food Habits and Nutritional Status in Southern Nigeria." *Journal of Tropical Geography* 49: 86–91.

Valentine, Theodore R. 1993. "Drought, Transfer Entitlements, and Income Distribution: The Botswana Experience." *World Development* 21, No. 1: 109–126.

Van Esterik, Penny. 1984. *Intra-Family Food Distribution: Its Relevance for Maternal and Child Nutrition*. Cornell University, Cornell Nutritional Surveillance Program Working Paper Series No. 31. Ithaca: Cornell University Press.

Victora, Cesar G., and J. Patrick Vaughan. 1985. "Land Tenure Patterns and Child Health in Southern Brazil." *International Journal of Health Services* 15, No. 2: 253–274.

———, ———, Betty Kirkwood, Jose Carlos Martines, and Lucio B. Barcelos. 1986. "Child Malnutrition and Land Ownership in Southern Brazil." *Ecology of Food and Nutrition* 18, No. 4: 265–275.

von Braun, Joachim. 1994. "Introduction and Overview." In: Joachim von Braun and Eileen Kennedy, eds. *Agricultural Commercialization, Economic Development, and Nutrition*. Baltimore: Johns Hopkins University Press, pp. 3–8.

———, Howarth Bouis, and Eileen Kennedy. 1994. "Conceptual Framework." In: Joachim von Braun and Eileen Kennedy, eds. *Agricultural Commercialization, Economic Development, and Nutrition*. Baltimore: Johns Hopkins University Press, pp. 11–33.

Walker, Thomas S., and James G. Ryan. 1990. *Village and Household Economies in India's Semi-arid Tropics*. Baltimore: Johns Hopkins University Press.

WHO. 1985. *Energy and Protein Requirements. Report of a Joint FAO/WHO/UNU Expert Consultation*. World Health Organization, Technical Report Series 724. Geneva: WHO.

World Bank. 1994. *World Development Report 1994*. Washington, D.C.: World Bank.

Wright, Eleanor Witte. 1985. "Food Dependency and Malnutrition in Venezuela, 1958–74." In: John C. Super and Thomas C. Wright, eds. *Food, Politics, and Society in Latin America*. Lincoln: University of Nebraska Press, pp. 150–173.

Wright, Thomas C. 1985. "Politics of Urban Provisioning in Latin American History." In: John C. Super and Thomas C. Wright, eds. *Food, Politics, and Society in Latin America*. Lincoln: University of Nebraska Press, pp. 24–45.

5

Food deprivation

Sara R. Millman and Laurie F. DeRose

Food deprivation is synonymous with individual malnutrition. Food deprivation will inevitably occur if there is food shortage or food poverty, but deprivation also affects individuals in households whose food supply would be adequate were it distributed evenly.

Our focus in this chapter is on variation along lines of age and sex. Women and children are often identified as "vulnerable groups" in the hunger literature. Accompanying discussions imply two distinct meanings for this term. Vulnerable groups may be *likelier* than others to experience hunger. In addition, *probable consequences* if they do experience hunger may be more serious for vulnerable groups than for others. Whole sets of households – for example the landless, those living in rural areas, those headed by women – are sometimes identified as vulnerable. Contrasts across groups of households were considered in chapter 4. We focus here on intra-household distribution of food. One of the questions this chapter will help answer is whether the burden of food poverty is shared equally among household members. Another is what types of individuals are likely to suffer from food deprivation in the absence of food poverty.

Causes of deprivation

Food poverty

Households that cannot secure control over enough food to meet the needs of all of their members are food poor. In chapter 4 we demonstrated that, although there are more food-poor households in food-short regions, food poverty is a significant problem in regions where food is adequate as well. Inequitable food distribution creates hunger even when supply is adequate.

The relationship between food deprivation and food poverty is quite similar to the relationship between food poverty and food shortage. Food deprivation is more common in households where there is food poverty, but food deprivation is a significant problem in households where food is adequate as well. Inequitable food distribution creates hunger even when supply is adequate.

Although these parallels are informative in conceptualizing the causes of the various levels of hunger, it is also important to recognize that distribution within – in contrast to across – households is governed by household economic conditions, discrimination, and understandings of nutrient needs. Food poverty is not likely to have the same kind of profound effect on the social rules and norms that govern the intra-household distribution of food that food shortage has on household entitlements. There are exceptions to this generalization that will be discussed below as we explore the causes of food deprivation and how likely they are, given household food poverty or the lack of it.

Discrimination

Discrimination is the most easily understood reason why individuals go hungry in households with adequate food. Discrimination results from some members being deemed more valuable than others. Although some discrimination is a household-level manifestation of inegalitarian attitudes pervasive in the society as a whole (e.g. women are less valuable than men, children are not fully human until after their first birthday, elderly people deserve higher honour), other discriminating behaviours reflect economically rational response to adverse circumstances.

For example, households can sometimes avoid food poverty by favouring wage-earners in the allocation of food. Protecting the productivity workers can enhance the total amount of available food, but household members who are not economically active are deprived relative to the income-generating members. Whether or not they are absolutely deprived depends upon whether their intake matches their nutritional needs. Even if their intake is less than their requirements, it still might compare favourably with a situation in which there was no discrimination in favour of earners. Since the 1970s, there has been reliable evidence that households in developing countries actually make these kinds of decisions (Gross and Underwood 1971; Pitt et al. 1990). There has been a resulting emphasis on improving total household income to make favouring preferred or productive members over others less likely to result in absolute deprivation.

Misunderstood needs

Food deprivation also results from misunderstood individual nutritional requirements. Individual need varies according to relatively stable factors such as basal metabolic rate and sex, but also with life-cycle variations such as age and maturation, reproductive status, and activity levels. Not just caloric needs but also micronutrient requirements vary among individuals within the same household, especially growing children and pregnant and lactating women in comparison with most other adults. Therefore, it is not surprising that households do not fully comprehend the nutritional requirements of all of their members or the synergism between nutrition and disease.

The ill have elevated and sometimes qualitatively different nutritional requirements that are another potential source of misunderstood need. However, disease also affects nutrition in ways unrelated to household decisions about food allocation. Even where sufficient and appropriate food is offered, unhealthy individuals are more likely to be food deprived because disease suppresses appetite and reduces absorption. Gastrointestinal diseases, in particular, impair the body's ability to absorb both micronutrients and calories.

Measurement of food deprivation

Only individual-level measurement can provide evidence of variations in food deprivation related to patterns of intra-household food allocation or other nutritional influences that affect people in the same household differently. Anthropometry is based on individual measurement and offers the largest body of evidence directly relevant to questions of age and gender variations in hunger. Unfortunately, comparability of such measures over the life cycle is limited.

The abundant anthropometric data on child malnutrition are very informative about comparisons across different groups of young children. We are less well situated to address possible discrimination against the elderly or between young children and others. Earlier chapters considered variation in the prevalence of child malnutrition across countries, or across socio-economic groups within countries, as evidence of variations in hunger along these lines. In this chapter, we use anthropometric data to show variations in the prevalence of childhood malnutrition by gender and across detailed age categories. The results both critically evaluate the notion that discrimination against girls is the rule and illustrate weaning as a crucial stage in children's malnutrition.

Data permitting comparison of dietary intake for individual members of a household are much less widely available. Where such data have been obtained, they must be combined with appropriately specified dietary requirements before we can reach conclusions about intra-household variations in dietary *adequacy*. In subsequent sections of this chapter we assemble comparisons of dietary adequacy by age and gender for a number of countries. Best represented is South Asia, in which discrimination against females in intra-household food allocation, as in other matters, is often thought to be widespread and extreme.

The data show that women in South Asia (as elsewhere) eat less than men in absolute terms. But women are also smaller and so need less food. The simple observation that certain people consume less than others is not necessarily evidence of discrimination. When consumption is expressed as a proportion of requirements, comparisons become more informative but also more complicated. For example, in India, Pakistan, and the Philippines, adult women who are neither pregnant nor lactating actually consume a higher proportion of their energy requirements than adult men (see evidence below), but dietary adequacy deteriorates sharply with pregnancy and lactation. The expected female disadvantage appears when average dietary adequacy for all women is compared with that for men. An explanation that relies on general discrimination against women in intra-household food allocation does not fit a situation in which those women who are neither pregnant nor lactating are better fed than men.

An additional complication, however, is that female requirements may *incorporate* gender bias. First, women's requirements are lower in part because women are smaller, and body size is partly determined by dietary intake. Thus, low intake is one cause of small size, which in turn is used to justify low intake. Second, most definitions of caloric requirements incorporate the assumption that women are less active physically than men. In situations where women undertake as much physical labour as men (or more), definitions of requirements incorporating this assumption underestimate their need. Finally, "the extra nutrition requirements of the pregnant women and lactating mothers require further acknowledgment" (Sen 1988). This argument is similar to the one developed earlier in this volume (chapter 2) with regard to the Hyderabad standard of weight-for-age by gender. Measurement of discrimination requires comparing intake with requirements, and estimates of requirements for both men and women need to incorporate realistic energy expenditures more carefully.

Indirect measures: Consequences and causes of hunger

Given the difficulties of obtaining and interpreting data on intake adequacy for large enough samples to support meaningful analysis, some researchers have relied on inference from data reflecting variables more or less directly affected by hunger itself. An arguably more important reason why indirect measures are sometimes favoured is that they measure consequences resulting from hunger; they measure hunger that is having an impact on people's functioning.

Disease and death are the most severe consequences used as indirect indicators of hunger. For example, Sen (1989) interprets a higher-than-usual ratio of female to male mortality rates (or even less directly, an unusually low proportion of females in a population) as evidence that females get less than a fair share of whatever food is available. Similarly, evidence of lesser access to health care for girls and women (Kynch and Sen 1983) is interpreted to reflect a pattern of gender discrimination that is likely to apply to nutrition as well. And if mortality goes up more sharply during a famine for one age/sex group than for others, it suggests that this group bears the brunt of the crisis (Watkins and Menken 1985).

Practices presumed to affect intra-household food allocation have also been interpreted as evidence of differential adequacy of diet for different members. For example, those who are served last at meals are often presumed to get less than a fair share (e.g. den Hartog 1973; Katona-Apte 1975; Senauer 1990). Similarly, it is often assumed that, when all family members eat out of a single dish, small children will be disadvantaged. Customs that reserve particular foods for certain members or forbid them to others are also cited as evidence of differences in dietary quality.

Use of such indicators of the causes or effects of intra-household food allocation are suggestive, but need further empirical investigation and confirmation. Customary preferential feeding of certain foods to males versus females may receive lip service, without shaping actual behaviours. Mortality is affected by causes other than nutrition, and differentials exist despite equitable distribution of food. Less access to health care (Kynch and Sen 1983) is in itself a potential explanation of female disadvantage in mortality that is sometimes taken as proof of sex bias in intra-household food allocation. Ratios of males to females in the population, in turn, are a function of gender-specific migration patterns as well as mortality differences. And *reported* gender ratios may also be affected by the tendency for censuses and other counts to miss people who are less visible, less valued, or viewed as less fully a member of the group. This last argument may apply most to Indian women who have migrated away from their natal villages into their husband's households, where they have relatively little status.

In sum, indirect evidence makes plausible the hypothesis that one group is less well nourished than another, but poor health outcomes can result from inadequate food, inadequate health care, or other forms of discrimination. To test the hypothesis that a group receives less food, it is necessary to focus more closely on either the balance of intake and requirements or its more immediate outcome, the individual's nutritional status.

Direct measures: Nutritional status and dietary adequacy

In the following sections we assemble both anthropometric and food-consumption data to explore issues of differential food deprivation and discrimination in intra-household food allocation by age and gender. The conventional wisdom in this area would tell us that females and children are likeliest to go hungry. For example, in the 1985 edition of UNICEF's annual report *The State of the World's Children,* Grant (1985: 37) asserts:

From girlhood to womanhood, the females of many societies are fed last and least. Malnutrition in girls is much more common than among boys and the fact that, on average, an American woman weighs approximately 25 per cent more than an Indian women is to be explained not by race but by food.[1]

Similarly, *Hunger 1992*, a widely circulated report on world hunger from the private voluntary organization Bread of the World, states (p. 23):

Pregnant and nursing mothers and children from birth to age five have greater nutritional needs than the rest of the population, but they are the least well-nourished people within low-income households in developing countries. Males tend to receive more and better food than females.

The conventional wisdom seems plausible and rests on a sizeable body of literature (for useful reviews see, e.g., Haaga and Mason 1987; Rogers 1983; Van Esterik 1984). However, the present review concludes that, while there are undoubtedly situations in which women and children are targets of discrimination in intra-household food allocation, this conclusion has been applied too broadly. Much of the widespread disadvantage of children and their mothers can be better understood in terms of childhood diseases and consumption patterns that restrict maternal intake during pregnancy and lactation, plus restricted access by females of all ages to health care, rather than as the result of food-distribution patterns that routinely discriminate against women and children.

Evidence

Gender differences

The United Nations Children's Fund (UNICEF) has assembled anthropometric data by sex for children in a total of 44 developing countries. Proportions of underweight were higher for girls in 25 countries and for boys in 19 countries. Many of the differences were so small that they could easily be due to sampling error[2] and should not be over-interpreted. Gender contrast in some countries, however, are substantial. The extremes of both male and female advantage are found in Africa. In Madagascar, 40.2 per cent of boys and only 33.5 per cent of girls were underweight in 1983–1984, for a *female* advantage of 6.7 percentage points. In a sub-national sample in Rwanda, 28.5 per cent of boys and 40.5 per cent of girls were underweight in 1982–1983, for a *male* advantage of 12 percentage points. Indonesia was the only other country with a gender difference of more than 4 percentage points: a 1987 study found 48.7 per cent of boys and 55.3 per cent of girls underweight. These data indicate that important gender differences in nutrition do exist in some populations. However, in many, rates of malnutrition are very similar for children and sometimes males are worse off.

Comparisons by gender of adult anthropometry are relatively rare but those present in the literature also do not show a consistent male advantage. For instance, a study of agricultural migrant workers in Brazil documented a marked female advantage on a range of anthropometric indicators. Although, on some of the indicators, women were clearly malnourished relative to the standard (Desai et al. 1980, as summarized in Hamilton et al. 1984 and reproduced in Kanbur 1991), men were more so.

A thoughtful review of African evidence for gender bias in anthropometry (Svedberg 1990) rejected the hypothesis of female nutritional disadvantage there and concluded that the different roles of African (as compared with South Asian) women provide them with greater control over food and enable them to avoid nutritional deprivation for themselves and their children. Proportions of children underweight, stunted, or wasted appeared to be slightly higher for males than for females in four studies. A larger set of studies gave average weights and heights of preschool children, schoolchildren, and adolescents by age and gender; ratios of these values to the medians of the National Center for Health Statistics (NCHS) weight-for-age and height-for-age standards were typically slightly higher for females than for males, implying a modest female advantage. For adults, average heights were compared with those in the tallest European populations. Men were further below the reference heights in 11 out of 17 sample populations, and women in only 4. Desirable weights for actual average heights were also calculated, and actual average weights were expressed as a ratio to these desirable weights. In all 17 populations, men were thinner, relative to weights defined as appropriate for their heights, than were women. As Svedberg notes, these data are not consistent with a pattern in which females receive less than their share of household food supplies.

Svedberg does not question that females in South Asia are less well fed than males there; in his interpretation of the African data, he focuses instead on reasons why a pattern presumed to hold elsewhere might not hold in Africa: the "relatively favourable and autonomous position" of women in Africa is taken as explaining the absence of female nutritional disadvantage.

The conclusion, that females are discriminated against in access to food, rests disproportionately on studies from South Asia. The social status of women is especially low in South Asia. Their economic activities are restricted and their income-earning potential is far lower than men's. They take resources (labour and bride-price) out of their natal households. These factors explain why females are perceived as less valuable than males in the region. The female ad-

138

vantage in life expectancy that applies in most countries is reversed in Bangladesh, Bhutan, Nepal, and Pakistan (World Bank 1992). Until recently, this has also been the case for India. A female *disadvantage* in mortality is generally explained in terms of preferential treatment of males, with poorer nutrition for females often specifically cited as a likely part of such a pattern of discrimination. We focus closely on evidence from this region because nutritional discrimination is likelier to exist and also likely to be more severe here than elsewhere.

Bangladesh

Chen et al. (1981), seeking to explain higher female than male mortality in Bangladesh, assemble both anthropometric and dietary evidence as well as data on morbidity and health-care utilization. This particularly thorough study was made possible by the extensive data collected in the middle of the 1970s as part of the ongoing research programme of the International Center for Diarrheal Disease Research, Bangladesh (ICDDR, B). Relative to the US-based Harvard standard of weight-for-age, 59.9 per cent of boys and 74.0 per cent of girls were identified as either moderately or severely underweight. Higher rates of underweight for girls than for boys in Bangladesh are also reflected in more recent data, although the contrast is less sharp: 64.8 per cent of boys and 67.8 per cent of girls were underweight in 1989–1990. Chen et al. (1981) find a similar pattern of female disadvantage in children's height-for-age, indicating that girls were more likely than boys to experience the stunting that reflects a long-term history of malnutrition.

This gender difference in nutritional outcomes of children is at least partly explained by discrimination against females in the allocation of household food supplies. Chen et al. (1981) show lower caloric intake for females than for males within every age group. In early childhood, recommended intakes are the same for girls as for boys, so the lower intakes of girls demonstrate a less-adequate diet. At later ages, requirements differ by gender in a manner affected by body weight, pregnancy and lactation, and physical activity. Chen et al. (1981) adjust for these differences (although cautioning that the adjustments are crude) and conclude that female diets are markedly less adequate than male at ages 0–4 and somewhat less adequate than male at ages 45+ (see fig. 5.1). Girls actually do slightly *better* than boys at ages 5–14. At ages 15–44 the contrast is dramatically affected by which adjustments are made: women of 15–44 appear to be disadvantaged relative to men when the additional caloric requirements

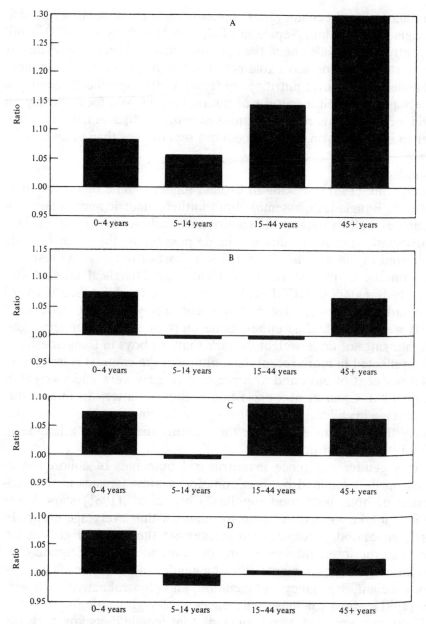

Fig. 5.1 **Bangladesh – ratios of male/female caloric adequacy by age groups: (A) actual; (B) adjusted for body weight; (C) adjusted for body weight, pregnancy, and lactation; and (D) adjusted for body weight, pregnancy, lactation, and activity (source: Chen et al. 1981)**

of reproductive status are included (panel C of fig. 5.1), but this disadvantage nearly disappears when adjustments for levels of physical activity are also included (panel D of fig. 5.1). When all adjustments are made, adequacy of the diet is quite comparable for prime-age adult men and women in this population. However, discrimination against females in food allocation is marked in early childhood and present to a lesser degree among older adults. The apparent parity in intake relative to need in the 15–44 age group may result in part from an underestimation of women's activity levels.[3]

India

A detailed examination of both anthropometry and food-consumption data from India's National Nutrition Monitoring Bureau (NNMB), provides little support for the expectation of general female disadvantage. The NNMB data are for large and representative samples of households in seven to nine states, depending on the round of their ongoing survey efforts.

Table 5.1 shows average caloric consumption, and adequacy of that average consumption, by state and requirement category. The standards with which the Indian dietary intake data are compared here are defined separately by physical activity level for both men and women, and individuals are assigned to activity-level categories corresponding to their occupations (NNMB 1981). The possibility remains that women's occupations are evaluated as involving less physical activity than they actually do. For instance, one might question whether a housewife in rural India really leads a sedentary life, although that is how she is classified (NNMB 1981)! None the less, this definition of dietary adequacy relative to activity-level-specific requirements is a serious attempt to eliminate the arbitrariness and possible bias implicit in applying the same requirements to all members of the same age and gender category regardless of their level of physical activity.

For the moment, we will focus on the gender comparisons in table 5.1, which start at age 13. Average consumption for females in most of rural India is less than they need. However, to justify a conclusion that females get less than a fair share, we should see caloric adequacy for males at a higher level, but females are less undernourished in most of the possible comparisons. At ages 13–16, girls receive a higher percentage of their requirements than boys in seven of the nine states covered. In the later teen years, females are less undernourished in all nine states. In adulthood, comparing males and non-

Table 5.1 **Mean caloric intake, expressed as proportion of requirements (Indian definition), by State and requirement category: rural India, 1975–1978**

Requirement category	Kerala	Tamil Nadu	Karnataka	Andhra Pradesh	Maharashtra	Gujarat	Madhya Pradesh	West Bengal	Uttar Pradesh	Requirement (calories)
Age (years):										
1	0.44	0.52	0.50	0.35	0.47	0.56	0.47	0.59	0.55	1,200
2	0.47	0.73	0.84	0.65	0.58	0.77	0.76	0.59	0.64	1,200
3	0.55	0.85	0.91	0.74	0.76	0.84	0.89	0.75	0.63	1,200
4 to 7	0.56	0.67	0.93	0.69	0.77	0.78	0.71	0.67	0.69	1,500
7 to 10	0.55	0.69	0.94	0.65	0.75	0.76	0.72	0.64	0.71	1,800
10 to 13	0.55	0.77	0.92	0.67	0.70	0.74	0.64	0.62	0.72	2,100
13 to 16 (boys)	0.48	0.69	0.91	0.60	0.67	0.70	0.62	0.69	0.81	2,500
13 to 16 (girls)	0.65	0.76	0.93	0.74	0.73	0.82	0.73	0.63	0.63	2,200
16 to 18 (boys)	0.53	0.66	0.79	0.67	0.63	0.69	0.68	0.62	0.74	3,000
16 to 18 (girls)	0.60	0.84	0.97	0.92	0.73	0.74	0.74	0.69	0.82	2,200
Adult males: sedentary	0.77	0.88	1.12	0.86	0.87	0.91	0.77	0.85	0.93	2,400
moderate activity	0.61	0.82	1.00	0.77	0.79	0.79	0.67	0.71	0.77	2,800
heavy activity	–	0.54	0.56	–	0.44	0.48	–	0.60	0.66	3,900
Adult females: sedentary	0.73	0.92	1.23	0.95	0.96	0.92	0.94	0.84	0.91	1,900
moderate activity	0.52	0.88	1.11	0.90	0.82	0.78	0.77	0.66	0.85	2,200
sedentary and pregnant	0.55	0.59	1.15	0.82	0.76	0.78	0.66	0.87	0.62	2,200
sedentary and lactating	0.45	0.65	0.87	0.68	0.69	0.68	0.73	0.58	0.61	2,800
moderate and lactating	0.50	0.67	0.67	0.80	0.55	0.74	0.90	0.55	–	2,900

Source: extracted and constructed from NNMB (1980), tables 27–44

pregnant, non-lactating females at the same activity level, 12 of the 18 comparisons show females consuming a greater percentage of their requirements. We return below to the question of nutrition during pregnancy and lactation.

The possibility remains that girls aged 12 or younger are under-nourished relative to boys of the same ages; since the NNMB does not publish food-consumption data separately by gender at these ages, the possibility cannot be tested with these data. However, the NNMB does provide anthropometry – a nutritional outcome indica-tor – by gender for children. The prevalence of underweight for both boys and girls is very high, but there is no female disadvantage.

Relative to the Indian growth standard, the anthropometric data given in table 5.2 show consistently and substantially higher rates of malnutrition for boys than for girls. This observation holds for rural children in all nine states covered by the NNMB, and for urban

Table 5.2 **Percentage of children aged 1–5 with weights less than 75 per cent of Hyderabad standard median weight-for-age (percentage moderately or severely malnourished)**

Region and period	Percentage malnourished			
	Male	Female	Average	Male – Female (= female advantage)
Rural India, 1979				
Kerala	39.7	25.2	32.5	14.5
Tamil Nadu	53.2	30.8	42.0	22.4
Karnataka	52.8	39.3	46.1	13.5
Andhra Pradesh	44.8	24.6	34.7	19.2
Maharashtra	49.5	39.9	44.7	9.6
Gujarat	49.6	40.3	45.0	9.3
Madhya Pradesh	61.8	52.6	57.2	9.2
Orissa	54.6	41.1	47.9	13.5
West Bengal	43.8	33.0	38.4	10.8
Uttar Pradesh	33.4	19.7	26.6	13.7
Average	*49.3*	*35.3*	*42.3*	*14.0*
Urban India, 1975–1980				
High income	12.0	10.1	11.1	1.9
Middle income	19.4	12.2	15.8	7.2
Low income	36.7	27.2	32.0	9.5
Industrial labour	38.6	30.0	34.3	8.6
Slum	52.1	39.9	46.0	12.2

Source: extracted and calculated from NNMB (1980, 1981, 1982).

children in each of five socio-economic status groups. However, as argued in chapter 2, the Indian standard of weight-for-age incorporates a bias in favour of males, and the apparent overall female advantage here is an artefact of this biased measurement (see also table 5.3).

Even though the apparent female advantage cannot be believed, variations in the pattern of gender contrast may still be meaningful. Most informative is the contrast across groups within India's cities. The groups are ranked from best-off to worst-off, as is apparent in the monotonic rising series of combined male and female proportions of underweight (column 3, table 5.2). Underweight rates for boys are clearly more sensitive to socio-economic status (SES) category than those for girls (compare columns 1 and 2, table 5.2). As SES increases, boys benefit more than girls. What appears (given the bias in the standard) as a 12-point female advantage among slum children diminishes to near-equality among children in high-income households. It is often assumed that any bias against females will operate more strongly in poorer households and thus that improvements in household economic situations will benefit females more than males. These data, however, suggest that preferential treatment for males, relevant to children's nutritional status, operates more strongly in households that have more resources. This finding is not inconsistent with other studies of gender bias among Indian children (Das Gupta 1987; Miller 1997). In fact, Miller's review of South Asian studies revealed a consistent pattern of greater gender bias within higher social groups and highlighted the fact that discrimination against girls among the wealthy may be hidden in the aggregate figures.

India's NNMB has applied both the NCHS and the Hyderabad standard to data for 1975 and 1989 (NNMB 1989). In comparison with the data shown in table 5.2, fewer states were covered, smaller samples were taken within each state, and urban areas were omitted entirely in the data subjected to this analysis. For these reasons, only summary figures for rural India are shown in table 5.3. As in table 5.2, female proportions of underweight appear lower than male, relative to the Hyderabad standard. In contrast, the proportions of underweight relative to the NCHS standard are virtually identical for boys and girls, at 61.9 per cent and 60.0 per cent, respectively, for the seven-state combined sample for 1989. When the presumably non-gender-biased NCHS standard is used, the female advantage that we see relative to the Hyderabad standard disappears. However, there is still no sign of the expected male advantage.

Table 5.3 **Percentage of children underweight, rural India**[a]

	Percentage underweight			
Standard and year	Boys	Girls	Combined	Female advantage
Hyderabad				
1975	55.5	44.2	50.3	11.3
1989	42.5	28.0	35.3	14.5
NCHS				
1975	71.6	71.6	71.6	0.0
1989	61.9	60.0	61.0	1.9

Source: extracted and calculated from NNMB (1989).
a. States covered are Kerala, Tamil Nadu, Karnataka, Andhra Pradesh, Maharashtra, Gujarat, and Orissa.

The Hyderabad standard, based on the anthropometry of the Indian élite, incorporates a bias against females and supports the point argued above that discrimination against girls occurs in relatively wealthy households. But this should not be generalized to Indian society as a whole.

Children's anthropometry is influenced by disease as well as by food intake, so we should not conclude from this evidence alone that girls' diets are as inadequate as boys' diets in India. However, to reconcile these data with a pattern of food allocation that discriminates against girls, one would have to postulate a female advantage in health strong enough to overcome the effects of less-adequate food intake. Medical anthropologists argue that males tend to be more vulnerable to physiological insult than females (Stinson 1985). On the other hand, preferential use of preventive and curative health care operates to the advantage of the preferred, in this case males. There is reason to believe that male children in some parts of South Asia do enjoy a favoured position with respect to these resources (see, e.g., Chen et al. 1981; Das Gupta 1987; Kynch and Sen 1983). The bottom line is that gender differences in anthropometry shown for India do not support the notion of substantial dietary discrimination against females in early childhood.

But anthropometric evidence is available only for surviving children. India has been known as one of the few populations in which males outlive females, and this reversal of the usual female advantage in life expectancy has itself been interpreted as evidence of poorer

145

nutrition for females. If this pattern persists,[4] however, these comparisons of food consumption and nutritional status suggest that the explanation does not lie in dietary but rather in health-care discrimination against females.

This conclusion must be qualified by highlighting the fact that not all of the states of India are covered by the data analysed here. Those omitted include some, such as Haryana and the Punjab, in which female status is believed to be the lowest. Kynch and Sen (1983) rank the states of India according to the ratio of females to males in 1981, interpreting lower values as indicating more-severe discrimination against females. By this measure, one might expect females to be worst off relative to males in Haryana and the Punjab and best off in Kerala and Orissa. Of the states covered by the NNMB data, the 1981 ratio of females to males was lowest for Uttar Pradesh, in which several of the gender comparisons within age and activity-level categories do favour males. State-level comparisons of male and female mortality patterns for 1969–1977 (Dyson 1989) also suggest that females may be more disadvantaged in Uttar Pradesh and the Punjab than in other Indian states.

Dietary-adequacy data from another source (M. Das Gupta and S. R. Millman, work in progress) are available for one of the two states in which analyses by both Dyson (1989) and Kynch and Sen (1983) suggest the status of women may be lowest. Figure 5.2 illustrates the age patterns of dietary adequacy for males and females in the rural Punjab. The curves intersect at several points, but adequacy is higher for females over much of the life cycle.

In this graph, female caloric adequacy figures during the reproductive ages are a weighted average of those for women who are pregnant, fully lactating, partially lactating (i.e. their youngest children are receiving other foods as well as breastmilk), or neither pregnant nor lactating. When these groups are disaggregated in figure 5.3, we see that dietary adequacy deteriorates sharply with pregnancy and further still with lactation. Male diets among 16–44-year-olds in this sample met almost exactly 100 per cent of their requirements. Therefore, reproductive-aged women who are neither pregnant nor lactating are actually better fed than comparable males. But women undergoing reproductive stress consume diets less adequate relative to need than men do. The slight female disadvantage we observe at ages 22–34 in the more aggregated data results from the high proportion of women at these ages who are either pregnant or lactating.

A similar pattern of deteriorating adequacy of the diet associated

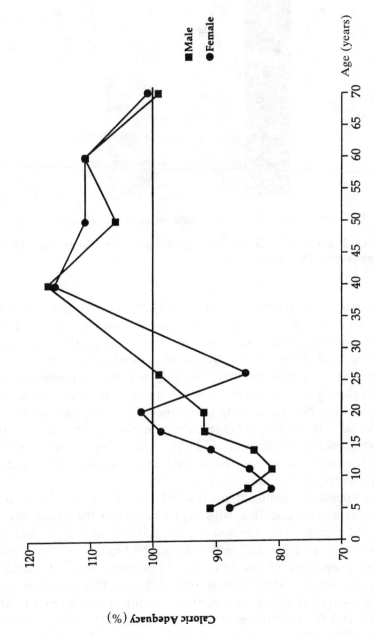

Fig. 5.2 Caloric adequacy of the diet by age and sex, rural Punjab: intake expressed as a percentage of requirements based on WHO/FAO recommendations (source: Das Gupta 1995)

147

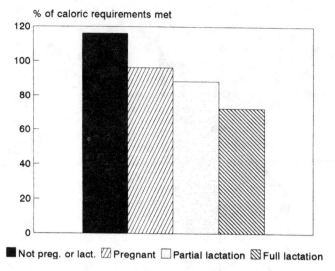

% of caloric requirements met

■ Not preg. or lact. ▨ Pregnant ☐ Partial lactation ◺ Full lactation

Fig. 5.3 **Caloric adequacy of the diet by reproductive status, women ages 16–44, rural Punjab (source: Das Gupta 1995)**

with pregnancy and lactation is observed for the multiple states of India covered in table 5.1. Pregnant women consume a lesser proportion of their requirements than women who are neither pregnant nor lactating, and in most states the situation during lactation is worse still. This pattern partly results from the increase in requirements during pregnancy and lactation. In some states, however, even *absolute* consumption declines during pregnancy; this is not just an insufficient increase. In others, average caloric intake is remarkably similar across women of differing reproductive status. At the best, we see increases that are less than proportionate to increased requirements, so that the average absolute caloric shortfall rises.

Women spend a significant portion of their lives subject to the nutritional stresses associated with reproduction, if they bear many children and if each child is breast-fed for many months. This pattern of severe undernutrition during pregnancy undoubtedly contributes to the high prevalence of low birth weight in India. Similarly, inadequate intake during lactation may limit breastmilk production and thus the growth of children for whom breastmilk is an important part of the diet. But the nutritional stress that women experience in their role as mothers does not affect only their performance of this role: their own health, their ability to perform other functions, and the quality of their own lives are also at stake.

Females appear to receive less than a fair share of household food supplies in some regions of India. The data suggest, however, that dietary discrimination against females does not apply to the country as a whole: the situation varies from state to state, across age groups, and across social classes. The only reliable generalizations are that females who are neither pregnant nor lactating take in more relative to their requirements than do men, but that, during pregnancy and lactation, women are at a strong disadvantage relative to men.

Variations in dietary adequacy by reproductive status, shown and discussed above for India, characterize other populations as well. In Pakistan and the Philippines, although the diets of pregnant and lactating women are sharply less adequate, women who are *not* pregnant or lactating also receive a *higher* proportion of their requirements than men of the same ages.

Pakistan

Table 5.4 summarizes the contrasts in dietary adequacy by age, gender, and reproductive status for Pakistan. Note first that, in childhood, before reproductive status becomes an issue, males and females are equally well fed. Average intakes for both genders are less than recommended, but there is no difference between the adequacy of the diet for girls and boys.

The only group that consumes, on average, more than the amount that the Pakistani government defines as its requirements, is that of adult women. No clarification was available as to whether this cate-

Table 5.4 **Caloric adequacy of the diet by age, sex, and reproductive status, Pakistan 1985–1987**

Age group	Sex/status	Caloric intake		
		Average	Recommended	Adequacy (%)
0–5 years	Male	1,166	1,300	90
	Female	1,169	1,300	90
6–15 years	Male	1,910	2,200	87
	Female	1,814	2,100	86
Adult	Male	2,532	2,900	87
	Female	2,237	2,100	107
	Pregnant	2,165	2,500	87
	Lactating	2,298	3,100	74

Source: Government of Pakistan (1988), as reproduced in Malik and Malik (1992).

gory refers only to non-pregnant, non-lactating women, or whether it combines them with the pregnant and lactating women whose status is also shown separately. If the latter is true, then intake by non-pregnant, non-lactating women must exceed their requirements by even more than is the case for the combined group. The less-extreme assumption is that "adult women" refers only to those who are neither pregnant nor lactating. In either case, the conclusion is clear: non-pregnant, non-lactating women are absolutely better fed than either men or other women. The adequacy of women's diets declines with pregnancy to a level comparable to that of men, and with lactation to a level considerably worse than that of any other group.

Philippines

For the Philippines, Garcia and Pinstrup-Andersen (1987) have calculated caloric adequacy ratios separately by age, gender, and quartile of household income. We reproduce their results in table 5.5. Gender differences are apparent that tend to favour males. However, the direction of this contrast is not consistent: except in the very

Table 5.5 **Caloric adequacy (proportion of requirements) for groups of individual household members, rural Philippines**

Gender	Age (years)	Income quartile				Total for entire sample
		First	Second	Third	Fourth	
Male	1–6	0.59	0.61	0.59	0.63	0.60
Male	7–12	0.65	0.70	0.70	0.69	0.69
Male	13–18	0.67	0.60	0.53	0.55	0.58
Male	19–39	0.74	0.80	0.75	0.73	0.75
Male	40–64	0.83	0.86	0.89	0.82	0.85
Male	65+	0.97	0.52	1.14	0.88	0.92
Female	1–6	0.52	0.56	0.55	0.59	0.55
Female	7–12	0.58	0.62	0.61	0.64	0.61
Female	13–18	0.58	0.62	0.60	0.63	0.61
Female	19–39	0.73	0.76	0.75	0.81	0.76
Female	40–64	0.78	0.88	0.93	0.76	0.84
Female	65+	0.90	0.90	1.09	1.11	0.98
Male (household head)		0.77	0.84	0.81	0.80	0.80
Female (spouse)		0.73	0.76	0.80	0.83	0.78
Pregnant or lactating women		0.68	0.72	0.68	0.72	0.69

Source: extracted from Garcia and Pinstrup-Andersen (1987).

poorest group, teenage girls receive a larger proportion of their requirements than do teenage boys. This female advantage is also apparent in the upper two income quartiles at ages 19–39 and in the middle two income quartiles at ages 40–64. The most consistent pattern of intra-household variation in caloric adequacy visible in these data is by age rather than by gender: the youngest children tend to receive a smaller proportion of their requirements than others, and elders are advantaged over others.

Although Garcia and Pinstrup-Andersen (1987) did not publish separate figures for non-pregnant, non-lactating women, it is clear that those who are pregnant and/or lactating have less-adequate diets than other women. Most of the women whose caloric requirements would be affected by their reproductive status are in the age group from 19 to 39; in every income quartile for that age group, the diets of pregnant and lactating women fall further short of their requirements than the diets of all women at those ages, because their caloric intake was virtually unaffected by their reproductive status, regardless of income level (not shown).

Other countries

In other countries, male dietary data are unavailable for comparison, but we can document a similar deterioration in the adequacy of women's diets associated with reproduction. McGuire and Popkin (1990) summarize results of studies on dietary intakes of women in developing countries. They show comparable data for non-pregnant, non-lactating, pregnant, and lactating women in four populations. Samples in these studies are not necessarily representative, and absolute levels shown cannot be extrapolated to national populations. Summary statistics are shown in table 5.6. All are consistent with the more detailed picture documented for India and Pakistan in showing that lactating women consume a less-adequate diet than the non-pregnant, non-lactating; all but Mexico also show a reduction in adequacy with pregnancy. Many additional studies, also summarized by McGuire and Popkin (1990), show values for caloric intake of pregnant or lactating women in developing countries far below requirements, but leave open the question of whether non-pregnant, non-lactating women in these settings do better.

In a population with high fertility and extended breast-feeding, women are likely to spend many years either pregnant or lactating. A significant nutritional disadvantage associated with these conditions may play an important role in the lives of most women. Insufficient

151

Table 5.6 **Percentage adequacy of women's diets by reproductive status**

Region	Status		
	NPNL[a]	Pregnant	Lactating
Rural Kenya, 1977–1979	84.0	First trimester: 67.2 Second trimester: 68.0 Third trimester: 59.0	76.1
New Guinea subsistence farmers			
Coastal	66.8	59.3	54.3
Highlands	98.5	83.9	82.0
Mexico	83.3	84.7	78.1

Source: McGuire and Popkin (1990).
a. NPNL: non-pregnant, non-lactating.

increases – or even restrictions – of intake with pregnancy and lactation, damaging though they undoubtedly are to women, do not signify general discrimination against females. Traditional concepts of low nutritional needs in pregnancy and lactation; loss of appetite or discomfort associated with eating large amounts of a bulky, grain-based diet during pregnancy; and beliefs that childbirth is likely to be more difficult if the baby is large and that dietary restriction to limit foetal growth is therefore beneficial, all may contribute to this pattern. However, if there were generalized discrimination against females in food allocation, it should be reflected in the food intake of females who are neither pregnant nor lactating and in child anthropometry.

Age

Young children

Comparisons of dietary adequacy over the range of ages commonly conclude that the youngest children receive less than their share. At first glance, this conclusion is consistent with data shown in tables 5.1 and 5.5, respectively for India and the Philippines, but the data require further scrutiny and clarification. If one-year-olds in Andhra Pradesh *on average* consume only 35 per cent of the energy they need, how do most of them survive? Infant and child mortality are higher than in the West, but not that high! The possibility that recorded intake of the youngest children is biased downward is borne out: the NNMB does not record breastmilk consumption. In populations that practise extended breast-feeding, mother's milk contributes significantly to the diet, well into (and even beyond) the second year of life. Assuming infant-feeding patterns are comparable to those in neighbouring Bangladesh, intake of one-year-olds in rural India may be understated by as much as 300 calories per day.[5] If recorded intakes of one-year-olds shown in table 5.1 are adjusted upwards by this amount, the resulting caloric adequacy figures are comparable to those at other ages. Even with this adjustment, Indian toddlers are getting fewer calories than they need. But whether they are getting less than their share of inadequate household food supplies is another question.

Assertions that infants and toddlers are targets of discrimination in intra-household food allocation may well be true in some situations. However, in at least some cases, the reason we have this impression is an artefact of data collection that omitted breastmilk.

Weaning
UNICEF has compiled evidence of detailed age patterns of children's underweight, wasting, and stunting for national populations throughout the developing world (Carlson and Wardlaw 1990). Regional patterns based on these national data are shown in figure 5.4a–c. While the prevalence of each nutritional problem varies from region to region, the age patterns observed are strikingly similar across regions. At each age, proportions of underweight are much higher in South Asia than in any other region, yet within each region we see a marked decrease in nutritional status (increase in underweight) from the first to the second year of life, followed by a more gradual decline from this peak.

All three indicators of nutritional status (weight-for-age, weight-for-height, and height-for-age) show a sharp deterioration during the second year. This pattern is replicated in almost every national sample as well as in the regional averages. Subsequent to this peak, the prevalence of wasting declines rapidly. Stunting tends instead to remain near the level of the second-year peak, in some cases increasing further.

Wasting, or low weight for height, reflects a current or recent nutritional crisis. Stunting, or low height for age, is the cumulative effect of a child's longer-term nutritional history, the result of either slow growth or uncompensated interruption of growth by a past crisis or crises. The marked peak in wasting in these data, and the rapid decline from this peak, show a transient nutritional crisis. In contrast,

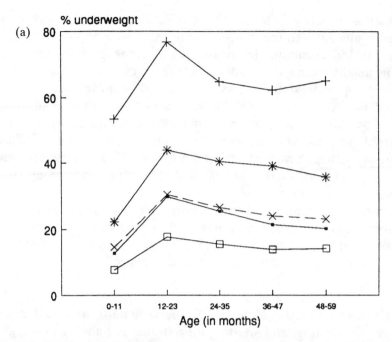

Fig. 5.4 **Patterns of (a) underweight (percentage below −2 standard deviations [SD] weight-for-age), (b) wasting (percentage below −2 SD weight-for-height), and (c) stunting (percentage below −2 SD height-for-age) by age in months, in Africa (•), South Asia (+), Rest of Asia (∗), the Americas (□), and global (×). Source: Carlson and Wardlaw (1990)**

the rapid increase and then stabilization of stunting shows the longer-term impact of this crisis on children's growth.

The crisis illustrated in these data is almost surely the process of weaning. The transition from breast-feeding to consumption of the regular family diet is likely to include increased exposure to disease through consumption of contaminated foods, especially where hygiene is poor. At the same time, the child is losing the immuno-logical protection previously available from breastmilk. If the onset of this transition is postponed too long, the child may be depending entirely on a supply of breastmilk that is no longer sufficient to meet its needs.

Additional difficulties may include the use of weaning foods that are too bulky for the weanling with a tiny stomach to eat in the nec-essary quantities, or that provide too little of certain nutrients even if enough is eaten to meet energy requirements. The combination of dietary constraint and an increased burden on infection encourages

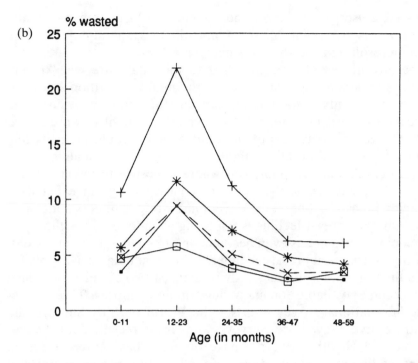

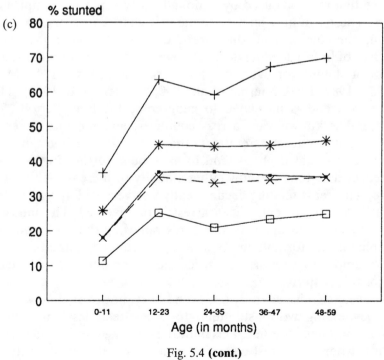

Fig. 5.4 **(cont.)**

repeated episodes of illness and weight loss. Children eventually outgrow this particular phase of nutritional vulnerability, but the stunting resulting from the crisis may persist.

The advantages of breast-feeding to the infant are well known: mother's milk is an optimal match to the infant's nutritional need, it has no opportunity to spoil before consumption, and it provides some protection against infectious disease while the infant's own immune system develops. Any loss of these advantages would be especially important where alternative infant foods are of poor quality, where sanitary conditions are poor, and where exposure to infectious disease is frequent. Thus, the depth of concern many have felt over declining breast-feeding in the developing world is understandable.

Fortunately, breast-feeding is *not* being abandoned throughout the developing world and is even becoming more common in some areas. Identifying trends in breast-feeding requires that data be available for more than one point in time. Only in the past two decades have such data become available for many developing countries. Three large-scale international survey efforts – the World Fertility Surveys, the Contraceptive Prevalence Surveys, and, most recently, the Demographic and Health Surveys – have obtained basic information on infant-feeding methods used by nationally representative samples of mothers. These can now be used to identify change over time.

Among the countries in which trend data are available, there are some cases of breast-feeding decline; however, they are outnumbered by cases of stability or even increase (Grummer-Strawn 1991; Millman 1986, 1987, 1990; Sharma et al. 1990; Trussell et al. 1990). The direction of trend is unrelated to geographic location. Periods for which trend is known vary across countries, and the one generalization about what differentiates the cases of decline and of improvement is that declines tend to have been further in the past: more-recent data tend to show either stability or increase. Thus, it is possible that breast-feeding decline really was very widespread in the past but has more recently been arrested or reversed. The international consumer movement of the 1970s opposing the promotion of commercial infant formula in the developing countries, and the associated attempts to support breast-feeding, probably deserve much credit for this pattern.

As a caveat to this generally optimistic story, however, élite women in the developing world still tend to breast-feed less than other women in the same societies. This pattern is reversed in industrialized countries, where the most-educated women are the most likely to breast-feed. Efforts to promote breast-feeding would do well to target these élite third world women since their behaviours may be emulated by others. If breast-feeding remains normative among women with high socio-economic standing – especially those holding modern-sector jobs – there is less chance that the current, apparently positive, trends in breast-feeding practices will be eroded by social change.

Elderly

Unfortunately, we know very little about whether the elderly are advantaged or disadvantaged by food-allocation practices within households. The data from the Philippines, presented in table 5.5, shows that those over 65, both male and female, consume a greater proportion of their estimated need than those at younger ages. The data from the rural Punjab in figure 5.2 show neither advantage nor disadvantage for the elderly.

From other scattered evidence about the intake patterns of the elderly, it is difficult to generalize. Intake is rarely compared with need, and households' food allocations to the elderly are likely to depend on their social standing in the society at large. Women in India experience increasing social status as they age; this pattern sharply contrasts with Western values, which ascribe social worth largely on the basis of productivity and therefore do not value the elderly as highly (Das Gupta 1995). But even in societies which honour their seniors, the elderly may receive inequitably small shares of household food. In Bangladesh, elderly members miss more meals than those in any other age group (Hossain 1987). In parts of India, widows typically eat only one meal per day (Katona-Apte 1975). The Indian elderly may also bear a disproportionate share of the burden when there is a food crisis (Harriss 1986). In Nigeria, the elderly observe food taboos that do not apply to the population as a whole (Bryceson 1989).

Discernible differences in the nutritional adequacy of elderly diets, where they appear, are likely to have multiple causes. Where older people are perceived to be either a burden or deserving of special honour, such valuations are likely to be expressed in appropriate food allocations. However, it is also possible that the intake needs of the elderly are *over*estimated, since their requirements decrease as their levels of physical activity decrease; this would provide an explanation of the pattern of reduced intakes among Filipino elderly, who may not suffer discrimination. In contrast, the increased nutritional needs of the elderly in poor health may go unrecognized and

157

lead to an underestimation of their needs, and underallocations. Illness may also interfere with appetite and cause them to underestimate their own need. Intakes by the elderly are also very much dependent on the form of food (e.g. soft or hard). Finally, the dynamics of household food allocation may be very different under crisis and non-crisis situations: the same elderly member who is accorded special honour on a regular basis may make extreme sacrifices if the survival of younger members is threatened during a food crisis.

Conclusions

Evidence reviewed in this chapter qualifies widely held beliefs about patterns of advantage and disadvantage in food allocation within households. We find little support for the notion that the youngest children tend to get less than a fair share of household food supplies: estimates of their food consumption have often been biased downwards by the omission of breastmilk from food-consumption data.

Rates of child malnutrition measured by caloric intake and anthropometry for boys and girls are quite similar in most countries. In household surveys, where both boys and girls fail to meet their nutritional needs, the usually small differences are as likely to favour females as males. These data do not only counter the notion that girls suffer hunger more than boys, almost everywhere: they contradict it even for India – the source of many of the studies that claim to document discrimination against girls in intra-household food allocation and from which broad geographic generalizations have been drawn. Although the sweeping generalization that Indian girls are discriminated against in the intra-household allocation of food is not supported by the data, there is strong evidence of such discrimination among Indians of high socio-economic status. The simple fact that the Hyderabad standard, which is normed from the anthropometric measurements of the Indian élite, incorporates gender bias would serve as adequate evidence of discrimination, even in the absence of village studies showing more discrimination against females in wealthier households.

We find that the generalization that adult women receive less than an equitable share of household food also requires qualification. For countries where women's intake data can be categorized by reproductive status, the diets of non-pregnant, non-lactating women are more adequate than those of men (though in most of these countries men and women are both undernourished). However, there is also compelling evidence of nutritional disadvantage for pregnant and lactating women in these same countries. Thus, even in populations in which women's status in general is low, we cannot assume that a simple pattern of gender discrimination in intra-household food allocation explains the poor diets of pregnant and lactating women.

The association of the most severe undernutrition with pregnancy and lactation implies that it really is in their roles as mothers that women experience the greatest nutritional stress. The particularly inadequate diets of women at these times compromises both their own and their children's health. This pattern calls for targeted interventions seeking to improve women's nutrition during pregnancy and breast-feeding. Most efforts to deal with hunger among women are oriented towards the nutritional stresses of reproduction; this orientation appears quite appropriate. A better understanding of the reasons for the declining adequacy of women's diets during pregnancy and lactation, however, may be necessary in order to develop interventions that will succeed in countering it. But, even with the available information, we conclude that these interventions need to do more than improve women's general status. The more favourable intakes of reproductive-aged women who are neither pregnant nor lactating argues against generalized discrimination and indicates that the nutritional needs during pregnancy – but particularly while breast-feeding – are either not well understood by women and their households or (for other reasons, including poverty) not addressed. The effect of other possible contributing factors, such as consumption of foods that are not sufficiently nutrient dense, might be countered by greater awareness of increased need as well.

Given that data on women's energy expenditures are generally unavailable, we must draw attention to the possibility that women's caloric needs are underestimated by common methodologies. The energy needs of women whose domestic and/or paid work is particularly arduous are especially likely to be underestimated. Interventions that target these women and improve understanding of their increased needs may also be appropriate.

If better information on actual energy expenditures in developing countries revealed higher energy needs for women (but not for men) than are commonly assumed, the adequacy of women's diets relative to need would be lower than indicated by the data presented in this chapter, while men's would stay the same. Non-pregnant, non-lactating women might continue to enjoy a relative advantage over men (but a smaller one), a picture of equitable food distribution might emerge, or men's diets might prove to be more adequate relative to need than women's – depending on the magnitude of the adjustment.

Finally, the detailed age data on children's malnutrition also pin-point the critical importance of weaning problems. Data permitting documentation of the weaning practices in different populations in comparable form are now available for the first time from the series of Demographic and Health Surveys (currently in Round III). Further investigation of weaning practices actually used in different popula-tions, and the consequences of these practices for children's health and development, should be a high priority.

Notes

1. There is little room for doubt that nutritional differences are largely responsible for the smaller body sizes of Indians compared with Americans. However, this comparison provides no information about women's food deprivation relative to men's within the same society. In fact, while, on average, Indian women weigh about 75 per cent as much as American women, the comparable figure for males is only 65 per cent (James and Schofield 1990). Indians are less well fed than Americans, but this particular comparison provides no support for the belief in a female disadvantage within India.
2. Since sample sizes are not given, this can be identified only as a possibility.
3. Chen et al. (1981) refer to the physical activity adjustment as "the most crude and difficult adjustment" which they make. They used labour force participation data from the 1974 census and WHO/FAO guidelines to calculate a 26 per cent average incremental require-ment for men aged 15–44 years; the increments for adolescents and men over 45 were slight. Adjustments for female work using the same set of recommendations yielded a 6 per cent increase for adult women, in part because of lack of quantitative information on the energy demands of household and home-based work.
4. The higher mortality of females in India may be a thing of the past; the more usual pattern of a female advantage in life expectancy seems to be emerging (Dyson 1989).
5. Brown et al. (1992) provide data on proportions of children still breast-fed and on amounts of breastmilk consumed by children by detailed age; they also cite previous analysis of the composition of breastmilk in the same poorly nourished population. These elements combine to define the caloric value of breastmilk consumption by detailed age of children in rural Bangladesh.

Works cited

Brown, Kenneth H., Robert E. Black, Stan Becker, Shamsun Nahar, and John Sawyer. 1982. "Consumption of Food and Nutrients by Weanlings in Rural Ban-gladesh." *American Journal of Clinical Nutrition* 36 (November): 878–889.

Bryceson, Deborah Fahy. 1989. "Nutrition and the Commoditization of Food in Sub-Saharan Africa." *Social Science and Medicine* 28, No. 5: 425–440.

Carlson, B., and T. Wardlaw. 1990. "A Global, Regional and Country Assessment of Child Malnutrition." *UNICEF Staff Working Papers* 7. New York, NY: UNICEF.

Chen, Lincoln C., Emdadul Huq, and Stan D'Souza. 1981. "Sex Bias in the Family Allocation of Food and Health Care in Rural Bangladesh." *Population and Development Review* 7, No. 1: 55–70.

Das Gupta, Monica. 1987. "Selective Discrimination against Female Children in Rural Punjab, India." *Population and Development Review* 13, No. 1: 77–100.

———. 1995. "Life Course Perspectives on Women's Autonomy and Health Outcomes." *American Anthropologist* 97, No. 3: 481–491.

den Hartog, A. P. 1973. "Unequal Distribution of Food Within the Household (A Somewhat Neglected Aspect of Food Behaviour)." *FAO Nutrition Newsletter* 10, No. 4: 8–15.

Dyson, Tim. 1989. "A Further Note on Trends in the Sex Differential in Mortality in India." Paper for informal session on sex differentials in mortality, IUSSP Conference, New Delhi, 1989.

Garcia, M., and P. Pinstrup-Andersen. 1987. *The Pilot Food Price Subsidy Scheme in the Philippines: Its Impact on Income, Food Consumption, and Nutritional Status.* Washington, D.C.: International Food Policy Research Institute.

Grant, James P. 1985. *The State of the World's Children 1985.* New York: Oxford University Press for UNICEF.

Gross, Daniel R., and Barbara A. Underwood. 1971. "Technological Change and Caloric Costs: Sisal Agriculture in Northeastern Brazil." *American Anthropologist* 73, No. 3: 725–740.

Grummer-Strawn, Laurence M. 1991. "Trends in Breastfeeding Behavior in Fifteen Developing Countries." Presented at the 119th Annual Meeting of the American Public Health Association, Atlanta, Georgia, November 1991.

Haaga, J. G., and J. B. Mason. 1987. "Food Distribution Within the Family." *Food Policy* 12, No. 2: 146–160.

Hamilton, Sahni, Barry Popkin, and Deborah Spicer. 1984. *Women and Nutrition in Third World Countries.* Praeger Special Studies. New York: Bergin & Garvey.

Harriss, Barbara. 1986. "The Intrafamily Distribution of Hunger in South Asia." Paper for WIDER Project on Hunger and Poverty; Seminar on Food Strategies, Helsinki, 1986.

Hossain, Mosharaff. 1987. *The Assault that Failed: A Profile of Absolute Poverty in Six Villages of Bangladesh.* Geneva: United Nations Research Institute for Social Development.

James, W. P. T., and E. C. Schofield. 1990. *Human Energy Requirements: A Manual for Planners and Nutritionists.* New York: Oxford University Press.

Kanbur, S. M. R. 1991. "Malnutrition and Poverty in Latin America." In: J. Drèze and A. Sen, eds. *The Political Economy of Hunger*, Volume III. Oxford: Clarendon Press, pp. 119–154.

Katona-Apte, Judit. 1975. "The Relevance of Nourishment to the Reproductive Cycle of the Female in India." In: Dana Raphael, ed. *Being Female: Reproduction, Power, and Change.* The Hague: Mouton, pp. 43–48.

Kynch, Jocelyn, and Amartya Sen. 1983. "Indian Women: Well-Being and Survival." *Cambridge Journal of Economics* 7: 363–380.

161

Malik, N. S., and S. J. Malik. 1992. *Reporting on the World Nutrition Situation: A Case Study of Pakistan (1976–1991).* Report prepared for the ACC/SCN of the United Nations. Islamabad, Pakistan: Economics Department, Quaid-e-Azam University and Washington, DC: IFPRI.

McGuire, J. S., and B. M. Popkin. 1990. *Beating the Zero-Sum Game: Women and Nutrition in the Third World.* Administrative Committee on Coordination/ Subcommittee on Nutrition, Discussion Paper 6. Geneva: ACC/SCN Secretariat.

Miller, Barbara D. 1997. "Social Class, Gender and Intrahousehold Food Allocations to Children in South Asia." *Social Science and Medicine* 44, No. 11: 1685–1695.

Millman, S. R. 1986. "Trends in Breastfeeding in a Dozen Developing Countries." *International Family Planning Perspectives* 12, No. 3: 91–95.

———. 1987. *Breastfeeding Trends in Eighteen Developing Countries.* Research Triangle Park, NC: Family Health International.

———. 1990. "Update on Breastfeeding Trends." In: R. S. Chen, ed. *The Hunger Report 1990.* Providence, Rhode Island: Alan Shawn Feinstein World Hunger Program, pp. 71–72.

NNMB. 1980. *Report for the Year 1979.* Hyderabad, India: National Institute of Nutrition.

———. 1981. *Report for the Year 1980.* Hyderabad, India: National Institute of Nutrition.

———. 1982. *Report on Urban Population.* Hyderabad, India: National Institute of Nutrition.

———. 1989. *Interim Report of Repeat Survey (Phase I) 1988–89.* National Nutrition Monitoring Bureau.

Pitt, Mark M., M. R. Rosenzweig, and Md Nazmul Hassan. 1990. "Productivity, Health and Inequality in the Intra-household Distribution of Food in Low Income Countries." *American Economic Review* (December): 1139–1156.

Rogers, Beatrice Lorge. 1983. *The Internal Dynamics of Households: A Critical Factor in Development Policy.* A report to the United States Agency for International Development. Medford, MA: Tufts University School of Nutrition.

Sen, Amartya K. 1988. "Family and Food: Sex Bias in Poverty." In: T. N. Srinivasan and Pranab K. Bardhan, eds. *Rural Poverty in South Asia.* New York: Columbia University Press, pp. 453–472.

———. 1989. "Women's Survival as a Development Problem." *Bulletin of the American Academy of Arts and Sciences* 43, No. 2: 14–29.

Senauer, Benjamin. 1990. "The Impact of the Value of Women's Time on Food and Nutrition." In: Irene Tinker, ed. *Persistent Inequalities: Women and World Development.* Oxford: Oxford University Press, pp. 150–161.

Sharma, R. K., S. O. Rutstein, M. Labbok, G. Ramos, and S. Effendi. 1990. "Trends and Differentials in Breastfeeding: Findings from WFS and DHS Surveys." Population Association of America Annual Meeting, Toronto, 1990.

Stinson, S. 1985. "Sex Differences in Environmental Sensitivity During Growth and Development." *Yearbook of Physical Anthropology* 28: 123–147.

Svedberg, Peter. 1990. "Undernutrition in Sub-Saharan Africa: Is There a Gender Bias?" *Journal of Development Studies* 26, No. 3: 469–486.

Trussell, James, Laurence Grummer-Strawn, Germán Rodriguez, and Mark Van-Landingham. 1990. "Trends and Differentials in Breastfeeding Behavior: Evidence from the WFS and DHS." Population Association of America Annual Meeting, Toronto, 1990.

Van Esterik, Penny. 1984. *Intra-Family Food Distribution: Its Relevance for Maternal and Child Nutrition*. Cornell University, Cornell Nutritional Surveillance Program Working Paper Series No. 31. Ithaca: Cornell University Press.

Watkins, Susan Cotts, and Jane Menken. 1985. "Famines in Historical Perspective." *Population and Development Review* 11: 647–675.

World Bank. 1992. *World Development Report 1992*. Washington, D.C.: World Bank.

6

Conflict as a cause of hunger

Ellen Messer

Throughout human history, conflict has been a source of hunger vulnerability. This chapter describes the range of ways in which "food wars" contribute to hunger, and the political and humanitarian efforts to limit food wars and why they succeed or fail. A "food war" is defined here as "the deliberate use of hunger as a weapon or hunger suffered as a consequence of armed conflict" (Messer 1990). Included in the concept are cases in which repressive measures and government policy meld to deny or restrict access to productive resources and income, as in the case of forced relocation in several African and Asian civil wars, and the discriminatory practices associated with legal frameworks or social practices of discrimination, such as apartheid in South Africa (Heggenhoughen 1995).

Scholarly, journalistic, policy, and humanitarian non-governmental organization (NGO) writings annually catalogue cases of food wars and consider the ways in which hunger vulnerability can be reduced after the wars have ended. They reported in 1994 at least 32 countries in which people suffered malnutrition, poverty-related limitations in their access to food, and acute food shortages as a result of armed conflict; and at least 10 more countries where hunger persisted in the aftermath of war, civil disorder, or as a result of conflict-related sanctions (fig. 6.1). Food relief and refugee organizations estimated that up to 50 million refugees and internally displaced persons needed food and other essential assistance, largely as a result of wars (WFP 1995).

Disruptions to food systems and economies also spill over to countries bordering conflicts. Refugees on the move away from con-

Africa

Western Africa	Eastern Africa	Southern Africa	Northern Africa
Burundi*	Eritrea	Angola*	Algeria*
Liberia*	Ethiopia	Mozambique	Ghana*
Niger*	Kenya*		
Nigeria*	Somalia*		
Rwanda*	Sudan*		
Sierra Leone*	Uganda		
Togo*	Zaire*		

Asia

Western Asia	Southern Asia	South-East Asia
Iraq*	Afghanistan*	Myanmar*
Turkey*	India-Kashmir*	Cambodia*
	Sri Lanka*	East Timor/West Irian (Indonesia)*
		Philippines

Latin America

Caribbean	Central America	South America
Haiti	El Salvador	Colombia*
	Guatemala*	Peru
	Mexico	
	Nicaragua	

Europe

Eastern Europe	Former USSR
Bosnia-Herzegovina*	Armenia*
Croatia*	Azerbaijan*
Serbia*	Chechnya-Russia*
	Georgia*
	Moldova*
	Tajikistan

Fig. 6.1 **Countries affected by food wars (by region): asterisks denote cases of active conflict where hunger has been used as a weapon (source: Messer 1996)**

flict and in search of food and fuel standardly devastate livestock, trees, and other natural resources on their way. Once forcibly settled or self-settled, they compete for land and other resources and affect local markets for food and livestock. Their additional demand for food and other essentials creates scarcities that drive up prices, while their need for cash drives down prices of livestock and other assets when they enter markets to sell them to get cash to buy food. Such distortions interfere with local coping mechanisms that ordinarily allow people to respond effectively to drought and avoid destitution, and turn food shortage into famine, as was the case in Western Darfur Sudan receiving refugees from the Chadian fighting (de Waal 1989).

After adjusting to a refugee or "relief" economy, borderlands may also find themselves destitute when the refugees go home, as has been the case for Malawian host areas when Mozambican refugees return to their native lands after years of residence. Conflicts therefore have an important regional dimension: they affect land use, food and commodity markets, livelihoods, and health, region wide, and in conflict areas it is usually wise to view hunger vulnerability of particular communities, households, and individuals in a regional context.

Food shortage related to conflict

The most obvious way in which armed conflict causes hunger is deliberate use of food as a weapon. Adversaries starve opponents into submission by seizing or destroying food stocks, livestock, or other assets in rural areas and by cutting off sources of food or livelihood, including destruction of markets in urban and rural areas. Land and water resources are mined or contaminated, to force people to leave and to discourage their return.

The deliberate use of hunger as a weapon is most evident in siege warfare and "scorched earth" tactics, but it is also evident where combatants commandeer and divert relief food from intended beneficiaries and keep emergency rations from affected civilian and displaced populations. Military interests appropriate both local and externally donated provisions for their own tactical advantage. A prolonged case in point is the Sudan, where the government in 1990 had sold grain reserves to fuel their military, but refused to declare a food emergency or allow relief into starving opposition areas. Both government and opposition forces created famine as a tool to control territories and populations, and restricted access to food aid (often by attacking relief convoys) as an instrument of ethnic and religious oppression (Keen 1994).

Food shortage ripples into the larger economy and extends over multiple years when farmers, herders, and others flee attacks, terror, and destruction or suffer reductions in their capacities to produce food because of forced labour recruitment (including conscription) and war-related depletion of assets. Ancillary attacks of disease, linked to destruction of health facilities, and hardship and hunger also reduce the human capacity for food production.

These factors set the stage for multiple years of food shortage, especially where conflicts interact with natural disasters such as multi-year droughts. Combined political–environmental disasters over several years produce the "complex emergencies" that now confront the international relief community. The World Food Programme, the International Federation of the Red Cross and Red Crescent Societies, other bilateral and multilateral relief agencies, and NGOs increasingly are called to respond to these emergency relief situations at the expense of peaceful development assistance aimed at increasing food production and livelihood in these same or other war zones (Maxwell and Buchanan Smith 1994).

Food-short countries

To identify populations that are food short because of conflict, a first step is to locate countries and their internal divisions experiencing warfare and to assemble local descriptive evidence of the ways in which the warring parties are using hunger as a weapon or otherwise destroying local food supplies or capacities to produce or access food. Not all peoples, regions, or communities are equally affected: some individuals always profit in times of shortage and conflict, and, in recent conflicts, asset-stripping of politically marginal peoples and the "relief-and-development" aid business have produced windfalls for certain groups (Keen 1994). Local and regional information about cultural (geographic, occupational, ethnic, religious, political) divisions can provide a guide for identifying predator "winners" versus preyed-upon "losers," pinpointing those groups most vulnerable to hunger within the region because they have suffered violent destruction or displacement or because they experience political or cultural barriers to emergency relief that need to be removed.

The extent of local damage can also be estimated by local information that can provide guidance as to whether destruction was total

167

or partial and what barriers will need to be overcome to restore (food production and other) economic activities. Food can be replaced, but poisoned water sources or land-mines quickly make land uninhabitable and prevent or endanger people's return. Complete asset-stripping of livestock, tools, and seed stocks means that such destitute populations require restitution of all factors of production to make economic recovery or food production possible. With agricultural and food assistance, annual crops can often be regrown the next season, but perennial crops may take years to re-establish.

Geographic distribution of food-short conflict arenas

Food wars take a large but selected toll in active and post-conflict zones (Messer 1996). In the 1990s in sub-Saharan Africa, food shortage prevailed in cases of active conflict, such as Angola, southern Sudan, and Somalia – where all sides in the conflicts used food and hunger as political tools – and in Rwanda, Burundi, and, to a lesser extent, Kenya – where those driven by violence from their homes faced both immediate and longer-term food shortages because they could not return to plant their crops.

As noted in chapter 3, the prolonged drought of 1991–1993 in southern and eastern Africa caused famine in politically unstable Mozambique but not in its more stable neighbours Botswana, Zimbabwe, and Kenya, which were able to organize effectively to respond to early warning signs of food shortage and to implement food relief.[1]

Unfavourable trends in food production continue to affect countries such as Ethiopia and Eritrea, where, years after their civil wars, landholding, water management, communities, and government infrastructures have yet to be rebuilt so that production and markets can be restored. Peoples in these countries are not starving, however, because they receive food aid and are sufficiently stable to distribute it.

Asian peoples in the former "rice-basket" countries of Cambodia and Myanmar similarly suffer food shortage as a result of prolonged conflicts, especially where military forces continue to use hunger as a weapon against opponents and to block food aid to affected areas. Siege warfare and armed struggle for control of relief food also characterize the new and old conflicts of western Asia, where residents of the Kabul area of Afghanistan remain on the brink of starvation despite donor efforts to rebuild agriculture, and warring peoples in the newly independent states of the former Soviet Union and Yugoslavia use food as a weapon.

Siege and starvation remain tools in the persistent conflicts in Sri Lanka, and food shortage confronts those whose lands and livelihoods have been destroyed in ethnic–religious and political-economic conflicts in India.

Iraq after the Gulf War faced the dilemma of inadequate internal food production after years of reliance on external food supplies exchanged for oil revenues. War-related destruction of infrastructure and economic trade sanctions harried any return to greater food self-sufficiency, while their leader refused to trade oil for essential food and medicines under UN mandate.

North Korea in 1996 offered a variation on the active conflict political theme. Although unfavourable weather sharply reduced grain availability, mid-year the government refused to declare a food emergency and the international community remained reluctant to send relief unless it could supervise its distribution to needy civilians, not to the military.

Interruptions in local food production also accompany internal conflicts in Latin America, especially in Colombia, Mexico, and Guatemala. Nicaragua and El Salvador are struggling to rebuild their economies and resettle otherwise military personnel after their bloody decades of civil war.

In the warring European states of the former Soviet Union and Yugoslavia, loss of livelihood accompanying the violence has left many entirely dependent on relief sources of food. Like their counterparts in developing countries, food shortage may be the situation of the affected countries, communities, households, and individuals for many years to come, as countries take years to rebuild agricultural infrastructure and productive populations after the wars end.

More positively, as a result of famine early warning and international response, the only places to have reported famines in recent years are the war-torn African and Asian zones of active or impending conflict. Only in conflict-affected areas does drought produce famine that kills. Post-conflict countries such as Ethiopia and Eritrea in the aftermath of war have experienced severe drought but not famine. They successfully appeal for, receive, and distribute food relief donated by the international community, but such external food sourcing is likely to be necessary for years to come.

Food poverty related to conflict

Conflict-related food shortages are also entitlement failures: people lose access to land, water, and other resources necessary for them to access food that they may or not grow themselves, and these deficits usually far outweigh losses in subsistence food production. To identify conflict-related food poverty, a straightforward approach is to locate zones of active and recent conflict, to chart gaps in productive and market capacities and in income, and to trace the relationships to recent conflict.

Food poverty related to conflict is most obvious in regions also experiencing food shortage, as described above. In addition, access to food may disappear as commerce is disrupted, either unintentionally (as in the Nigerian civil war, where all trucks were diverted to the war effort) or intentionally (as where Angolan rebels deliberately destroyed markets). In the Sudan, ethnic peoples such as Dinka and Nubians suffered food poverty as they were systematically stripped of livestock and other wealth, rendered destitute, and displaced, by rival groups armed by the government, which also profited from their demise (Keen 1994).

Entitlements also are reduced where individuals can no longer migrate to wage schemes or send remittances. Rural households suffer where they are cut off from cities, markets, and networks that ordinarily provide them with livelihoods or buffers against scarcity. Rural pastoralists suffer special hardship where mobility is circumscribed, traditional pasturage ranges are devastated, and local grazing zones undermined by resultant overgrazing. Precipitous drops in the price of livestock remove household buffers against shortfalls and eliminate assets available to invest in their future food supply. The end of manure to nurture agriculture or of income to purchase seed can lead to longer-term deterioration of crop production and income.

Similarly, people cannot risk holding crops over multiple seasons as insurance; the "safer" strategy of converting them immediately into mobile resources may cause them to lose income as well as future food security. As a general rule, coping mechanisms are undermined by violence and social disruption.

Rural populations also suffer increased hunger vulnerability where their own urban or other refugees, fleeing conflict or related hunger, retreat to the countryside, where they try to live off the land. Resultant changes in the local units of food production, distribution, and consumption, in response to these wartime additions, in most cases do not manage to feed all the new mouths, nor does additional production usually suffice to replace losses in marketed food.

Distribution of conflict-related food poverty

Unfortunately, aggregate statistics (country-level estimates are usually the only data available) cannot indicate the extent or precise distribution of shortfalls in food and livelihood. Market and other entitlement losses may far exceed crop losses as multiple and diversified sources of income shrink and people lack exchange entitlements for food. They also have consequences for local, household, and individual food security far into the future.

After the wars, communities decimated and depopulated by physical and human losses can remain underproductive and hungry for years, as food wars and the conditions leading up to them remain a legacy of armed conflict that is not easily remedied without outside assistance. Individuals, households, and communities must regain access to land, water, and other sources of livelihood, and human resources and social infrastructure must somehow recover. Communities in many cases must be re-formed, especially where areas have experienced complete or selective depopulation. Production and markets must be re-established, so that goods can flow and livelihoods rebound.

During prolonged warfare, whole generations may be conscripted into the military; with no other schooling, they must later be socialized into peacetime occupations if they are not to revert to violence and brigandage as a source of entitlements. In the African conflicts of Mozambique, Liberia, and Sierra Leone, destruction of kinship units was a deliberate military strategy to remove intergenerational ties and community bonds and create new loyalties – to the military. These grown youths now need sustenance, and basic and specialty education, if they are to contribute to a peacetime economy and society, and to general food security. After decades of civil war, these countries also lack skilled agricultural, social, and health professionals to speed recovery. They require agricultural, health, educational, and economic services to rebuild societies, as well as physical infrastructure such as agricultural works, transport and communication lines, and market-places destroyed in the wars.

There is little evidence specifying what points of resilience or sociocultural mechanisms help war-destroyed societies and food systems to "bounce back" after conflict.

Food deprivation related to conflict

Even where food resources are available from domestic or external (relief) sources, access is selective. As already noted in the case of Sudan, governments selectively deny access to opposition groups, and opposition leaders reciprocate by denying food to government-controlled forces and towns, where possible. In addition, certain members of households and communities have less access to regular food sources or emergency rations because they are relatively powerless as a result of their age or gender status. These include women, children, and the elderly, who are the most frequent victims of hunger in food wars, because they are left behind when active males migrate in search of food or are commandeered into military service where they are fed. Women often are forced to give up local assets (land, seeds), go without extra labour (especially of absent males), suffer lack of protection (against violence, as local community moral and social structures are destroyed), and enjoy less health care. Both women and children suffer disproportionately from illness, where malnutrition and destruction of health-care services render them more vulnerable, especially if, in the end, they are forced to flee in search of survival.

Children lose access to material and social resources at all social levels and are therefore more at risk of malnutrition, illness, and death. The most immediate and dramatic victims of hunger and war tend to be children, who die in great numbers of malnutrition-related illness; in Somalia in 1992, some estimate that up to 90 per cent of children under five died. It is a truism that governments at war invest fewer resources in child welfare: they favour military expenditures, and international assistance and investment (especially under conflict conditions) do not make up the deficit. UNICEF attempted to measure these investments by assessing which countries are least likely to meet World Summit for Children goals for improved child survival by the end of the decade. In their sample, those least likely to meet them are all "countries currently or recently affected by war or internal strife: Angola, Burundi, Haiti, Lesotho, Liberia, Mozambique, Rwanda, Somalia, Sudan, and Zaire" (Mason et al. 1996).

War-related refugee and displaced persons who have fled to situations that lack sanitation, water, and health services are especially susceptible to respiratory and gastrointestinal disorders that threaten lives (Winter 1995). Children are, in addition, exceptionally vulnerable to micronutrient deficiencies that generally characterize emergency food rations, which supply predominantly calories through cereals, legumes, and edible oils. Women are special victims of both violence and hunger in refugee settings, where male thugs often control distribution of emergency rations.

Everyone is rendered more vulnerable to malnutrition as a result of higher levels of illness, a by-product of the deliberate or accidental destruction of health services and underinvestment in health programmes that accompanies war. The most vulnerable members of society are also more at risk of hunger as a result of underinvestments in food security and development because of relatively high military or defence expenditures. In most cases of conflict, the longer-term economic and fiscal burden of war appears far more costly in terms of human lives than is direct killing (Macrae and Zwi 1994).

The hunger costs of sanctions

Another source of conflict-related hunger is the economic sanctions that are meant to forestall or replace military actions and bring about political change. Although essential foods and medicines are explicitly excluded from embargo, the poor have less access to nutrition and medicine because cut-backs in petroleum and other items essential for moving food, and higher prices for now-scarcer foods and medicines, are magnified by their reduced earning power in a failing economy. Those delivering humanitarian aid have still not found a good way to reach those most disadvantaged by sanctions. Significant excesses in child mortality in Haiti and Iraq have been attributed to the sanctions levied against Haitian military leaders (who seized power from President Aristide in 1993) and the Iraqi ruler, Saddam Hussein, in the aftermath of the Gulf War. In the latter case, journalists reported that an excess 500,000 Iraqi children have died in the five years that sanctions have been imposed. In each case, food and health care became unaffordable for the lower economic classes of population. Critics of this humanitarian argument against sanctions counter that it is not the sanctions but the repressive regimes that are largely to blame. Underlying political economic and sociocultural conditions also contribute in additional ways to conflict-related hunger.

Underlying conditions

Food wars tend to be fuelled by the quiet or active violence of preceding conditions – colonial or subsequent land regimes that favour social inequalities, commercial over subsistence production, and export agriculture that benefits landholders over workers or encourages highly specialized commodity production that is extremely vulnerable to world market fluctuations. The collapse of the coffee economy in Rwanda, as a case in point, left local cultivators vulnerable to hunger and hopelessness, and also ripe for political manipulation into violence that led to more widespread hunger and destruction (Uvin 1996).

Government allocations to military, rather than social, expenditures have led to national societies characterized by limited basic skills, food insecurity, malnutrition, and ill health as well as discontent, violence, and despair (Sivard 1994; Stewart 1993; Smith 1994). Military preparedness in this way creates conflict potential and constitutes one of the underlying causes of food insecurity that can lead to war.[2]

International donors sometimes exacerbate such underinvestments by demanding more fiscal responsibility from governments, a directive that policy makers often translate into lower levels of expenditures for food subsidies, health programmes, and education programmes. Critics of economic-adjustment programmes see them as a potential source of hunger and conflict. Specific indices of government social and military expenditures, however, reveal a mixed picture and are not in themselves good guides to pockets of hunger, although conflict potential may be linked to indicators of underdevelopment (Stewart 1993; Smith 1994).

One proposed solution to the conflict potential of differential underdevelopment is for international donors and governments to target zones experiencing economic hardship with additional economic assistance. Efforts may be ineffective because, among other reasons, the underlying conditions are more cultural and psychological than political-economic, and the hungry are those out of power suffering discrimination or overt violent attacks. To locate and intervene, in these special instances of disadvantage and underprivilege, then becomes the task of humanitarian rather than development aid, although the two increasingly are interlinked to limit hunger in cases of conflict and its aftermath.

Humanitarian and political principles and institutions limiting conflict-related hunger

Conflict-related hunger in the shadow of the post-World War II United Nations is both counted and countered by UN intergovernmental and other bilateral and international agencies. Every society has traditions that restrict permissible violence against fellow human beings, the environment, and livelihoods. They usually limit application of these principles, however, to those of their own cultural kind.

By contrast, international human rights and humanitarian covenants, which specifically provide for feeding of civil populations in international and intranational wars, are meant to be universal. The second, third, and fourth Geneva Conventions (1949) and Additional Protocols (1977) provide international guidelines to combatant parties for meeting essential humanitarian needs and ensuring basic subsistence rights of civilian populations experiencing armed conflict.

The International Federation of the Red Cross–Red Crescent Societies and NGOs, in accordance with these principles, intervene to move food into zones of armed conflict. Following humanitarian principles adopted by the United Nations, the UN High Commissioner on Refugees, the World Food Programme, UNICEF, and the United Nations Development Programme (UNDP) also are engaged with limiting destructive hunger due to war and promoting survival. International NGOs, such as CARE, Catholic Relief Services, Concern, Save the Children, and Médecins sans Frontières ("Doctors Without Borders"), along with regional NGOs, also move food into conflict and refugee areas. They also try to assist the restoration of order and to rebuild while providing food after the wars. All follow the Human Rights principles expressed in the UN Charter and Universal Declaration of Human Rights that declare that food is a basic human right and a principal component of the universal human right to life.

International legal instruments, such as the International Conference on Nutrition World Declaration and Plan of Action for Nutrition (1992) and the Vienna Declaration on Human Rights (1993), support the principle that food should never be used as a political tool nor hunger as a weapon. They provide a reference point and standard for action for the United Nations, its member states, and its agencies.

A third set of principles protects the refugee victims of conflict who have crossed borders or are otherwise stateless and therefore beyond protection of any UN member.

A principal concern for all those using these legal principles to justify food relief interventions is to handle food flows in ways that reach the neediest victims and do not further nourish the oppressors, combatants, and conflict. Even allegedly "successful" multilateral efforts to feed the hungry on both sides of the conflict, such as Operation Life Line in the Sudan in 1989, have been criticized as prolonging the war effort by providing recognition and legitimacy to insurgents and giving everyone time for a respite that encouraged them to fight on.

Also criticized for prolonging conflict are food relief operations implemented by "military humanitarianism." In very recent conflicts, large-scale food aid has been delivered by an international military force, a solution favoured in circumstances where logistics and security concerns make it unlikely that civilian operations can deliver food successfully, as in Iraqi Kurdistan, Somalia, Bosnia, and Rwanda. But use of the military in support of humanitarian action, such as movement of food into zones of armed conflict, also has been criticized for its war-prolonging potential. None of these operations have met humanitarian needs very successfully, and the combined military and food dimensions of aid intensify armed aspects of conflict by providing food, employment, income, and opportunities for further pilferage (Duffield 1994).

Another concern is to use relief in a manner that can help restore livelihoods and food security. Food-for-work theoretically is the relief mode of choice, especially in circumstances where people need food and income and where public works, such as land and water management, must be rebuilt. In conflict, or post-conflict, situations, however, the logistics of food-for-work may be impossible or inadvisable for at least two reasons: first, social infrastructure is needed to organize labour and communities, where none may exist; second, the most needy may not be fit for work, and may be excluded from food distributions if labour participation is the criterion for receiving food. These constraints, which have been described recently in the case of Ethiopia, are specific examples of the difficulties of calculating and remedying the multidimensional and longitudinal "hunger" costs of war (Davies 1994; Maxwell and Lirensu 1994).

Measuring the "hunger" costs of conflict

Conflict takes its multi-year toll in country-level food production and imports; in community- and household-level livelihoods; and in individual nutrition, health, and longevity. A simple but undiscriminating method of calculating the numbers of people affected by "food wars" is to sum the numbers of people living in war-affected countries. This was the method followed in earlier World Hunger Program *Hunger Report(s)* from 1988 (Kates et al. 1988). As has been pointed out here, however, this procedure greatly overestimates the numbers of those actually starving, disentitled, or otherwise deprived of nutrition and fails to distinguish the parallel economy that accompanies conflict and relief efforts (Duffield 1994; Keen 1994). It also misses the numbers who have fled the conflict to neighbouring zones or the economic distortions introduced into adjacent territories by additional people, by sources of (relief) income, and also by economic downturns due to disruptions in trade or sanctions. The following sections review the limited number of models and measures suggested to account better for damage leading to hunger, which might also be used to establish priority needs for future relief and development efforts.

Losses in food production

The food and hunger costs of war are sometimes tallied as estimated losses in food production. One study (Stewart 1993), which looked at 16 wars in the developing world over the 1970s and 1980s, found that food production per capita fell in all but two of the countries concerned, and noted falls of 15 per cent or more in Cambodia, Nicaragua, Sudan, Angola, and Mozambique.

Another recent analysis of food-production trends in countries experiencing warfare estimated that food-production growth losses on account of conflict over the 1970s to 1990s were, on average, almost 3 per cent per year in war-torn African countries (Messer et al. 1997). The FAO country-level data on which these estimates are based are not extremely reliable: especially in times of crisis, data collection and reporting techniques may lack accuracy, miss within-country variations, and not take into account significant contributions of the informal economy. Moreover, the impact of conflict on food production is complex, and hard to separate from other factors. But even so, the data strongly suggest (expected) downward trends due to destructive synergisms between armed conflict and bad weather, human malnutrition and illness, social disruption, and volatile commodity prices and availability that jointly impact on food production, distribution, and consumption.

These estimates do not touch on additional economic impacts of losses in food production, such as the foreign-exchange costs of food imports during wartime or the higher risks and costs of transportation. Someone (in recent times, usually external humanitarian organizations) must bear these costs for there to be food aid to make up the shortfalls in conflict and post-conflict areas, or the populations go hungry. There are also multiplier effects of crops not grown because agricultural services disappeared or inputs were not available for lack of local funds or state-level foreign exchange, or because of sanction-related import restrictions. These translate into growing deficits in local, regional, and state income and magnify losses in entitlements to food.

Entitlement losses

Losses in material and infrastructural goods that create income can be calculated roughly by estimating and adding specific items and then "guesstimating" multiplier effects. These numbers can then be compared with those arrived at by estimating probable output (growth) in the absence of war (Green 1994: 41). The second method is a general economic case of the specific food-output growth calculation suggested in the preceding section.

More directly, household-level hunger costs can be measured as lowered per capita income or entitlements to access food. On this measure, among countries at war in the 1980s, Mozambique, Liberia, Nicaragua, Afghanistan, Guatemala, and Uganda were the worst off, and their poor performance was almost certainly war related. Their capital and human resource base had been depleted. Sivard (1994), among others, has sought to measure the costs of war indirectly by comparing military against social expenditures at a country level.

Overall, the inestimable losses in crops and other components of the gross domestic product, plus social expenditures (human capital investments), have been judged to be far greater than military expenditures. But analysts are just beginning to measure them. "Human capital" losses in a vicious cycle affect productivity, nutrition, and life quality. The costs of war, carrying associated risks of food insecurity, endure far into the reconstruction and rehabilitation period. But economists have barely begun the calculations.

Losses in human life

Excess deaths due to conflict include the numbers due to active violence and the greater numbers due to passive violence of malnutrition, illness, and social disruption. Loss of life associated with

hunger has been observed to be most severe among those populations specifically preyed upon by oppressive regimes, as in the
case of indigenous peoples in Guatemala, traditional African ethnic
groups such as the Dinka and Nubians in the Sudan, and competing
political and ethnic groups in Angola, Mozambique, and Ethiopia
(Dergue).

Excess child deaths due to hunger and violence run into the millions. UNICEF calculated that over 1.5 million had been killed, over
4 million physically disabled, and over 12 million rendered homeless
in conflicts over the previous decade (UNICEF 1989; Grant 1994).
Restoring hope, skills, and social support for such passive victims
of conflict remains the significant challenge for building future food
security.

Conclusions

In summary, "famine that kills" in recent times is almost always
associated with conflict, either directly or indirectly. Although the
costs of conflict are usually measured in direct military expenditures
and violence-related human mortality, to these numbers must be
added the direct output losses and multiplier effects of reduced
demand for goods and services and for domestic and foreign investments foregone because of lack of peace and political-economic stability. More than from direct military encounter, civilian deaths occur
from the synergisms between stress, malnutrition, and illness that are
heightened by forced migration and social disintegration.

Notes

1. In 1995–1996, after two bumper harvests, Ethiopia for the time being was no longer food
   short, although problems of food security and malnutrition persist.
2. Security measures in rare instances also include food-security measures, as in Israel, which
   made special efforts to protect internal food supplies in case of attack.

Works cited

Davies, S. 1994. "Public Institutions, People, and Famine Mitigation." *IDS Bulletin*
25, No. 4: 46–54.
de Waal, Alexander. 1989. *Famine That Kills: Darfur, Sudan 1984–1985.* Oxford:
Clarendon Press and New York: Oxford University Press.
Duffield, Mark. 1994. "The Political Economy of Internal War: Asset Transfer,
Complex Emergencies, and International Aid." In: J. Macrae and A. Zwi, eds.
War and Hunger. London: Zed Books, pp. 50–70.

Grant, James. 1994. *The State of the World's Children 1994*. New York: UNICEF.

Green, Reginald H. 1994. "The Course of the Four Horsemen: The Costs of War and Its Aftermath in Sub-Saharan Africa." In: J. Macrae and A. Zwi, eds. *War and Hunger*. London: Zed Books, pp. 37–49.

Heggenhougen, K. 1995. "The Epidemiology of Functional Apartheid and Human Rights Abuses." *Social Science and Medicine* 40, No. 3: 181–184.

Kates, Robert, R. S. Chen, T. Downing, J. X. Kasperson, E. Messer, and S. Millman. 1988. *The Hunger Report: 1988*. Providence, Rhode Island: Brown University World Hunger Program.

Keen, David. 1994. "The Functions of Famine in Southwestern Sudan: Implications for Relief." In: J. Macrae and A. Zwi, eds. *War and Hunger*. London: Zed Books, pp. 111–124.

Macrae, Joanna and Anthony Zwi, eds. 1994. *War and Hunger. Rethinking International Responses to Complex Emergencies*. London: Zed Books.

Mason, John, Urban Jonsson, and Joanne Csete. 1996. "Is Childhood Malnutrition Being Overcome?" In: E. Messer and P. Uvin, eds. *The Hunger Report: 1995*. Amsterdam: Gordon & Breach, pp. 157–184.

Maxwell, Simon, and Margaret Buchanan Smith, eds. 1994. *Linking Relief to Development*. Institute of Development Studies, University of Sussex Bulletin 25, No. 4.

———, and A. Lirensu. 1994. "Linking Relief and Development. An Ethiopian Case Study." *IDS Bulletin 25*, No. 4: 65–76.

Messer, Ellen. 1990. "Food Wars: Hunger as a Weapon of War." In: Robert Chen, ed. *The Hunger Report: 1990*. Providence, Rhode Island: Brown University World Hunger Program, pp. 27–36.

———. 1996. "Food Wars: Hunger as a Weapon of War in 1994." In: E. Messer and P. Uvin, eds. *The Hunger Report: 1995*. Amsterdam: Gordon & Breach, pp. 19–48.

———, M. Cohen, and T. Marchione. 1997. *Food From Peace*. Report to IFPRI 2020 Vision for Food, Agriculture, and the Environment. Washington, D.C.: IFPRI.

Sivard, Ruth. 1994. *World Military and Social Expenditures*. Leesburg, Virginia: WSME.

Smith, D. 1994. *War, Peace, and Third World Development*. Occasional Papers 16. Oslo: International Peace Research Institute, Human Development Report Office.

Stewart, Frances. 1993. *War and Underdevelopment: Can Economic Analysis Help Reduce the Costs?* Oxford: International Development Centre.

UNICEF. 1989. *Children on the Frontline: The Impact of Apartheid, Destabilization and Warfare on Children in Southern and South Africa*. Third edition. New York: UNICEF.

Uvin, Peter. 1996. "The State of World Hunger." In: E. Messer and P. Uvin, eds. *The Hunger Report: 1995*. Amsterdam: Gordon & Breach, pp. 1–18.

WFP (World Food Programme). 1995. *Annual Report of the Executive Director 1994: Linking Relief to Development*. 39/4. Rome: CFA.

Winter, R. 1995. "The Year in Review" In: US Committee for Refugees, ed. *1995 World Refugee Survey*. Washington D.C.: Immigration and Refugee Services of America, pp. 2–7.

7

Conclusions

Ellen Messer

In 1995, hunger numbers indicated that 800 million people were food poor, tens of millions suffered iron, iodine, and vitamin A deficiencies, and millions were food short because conflict made it impossible for market or relief food to compensate for local shortfalls. The hunger numbers and profile (Uvin 1996), viewed against the findings of the foregoing chapters, suggest the following generalizations about where the hungry are located and certain themes for intervention to prevent and relieve nutritional suffering.

Patterns of risk

Food shortage

Those most at risk of food shortage tend to be located in conflict zones, where food cannot reach them. Weather and hazardous climatic or environmental conditions are less important than politics influencing food production and distribution. Active and post-conflict zones suffering food shortage predominate in sub-Saharan Africa and, to a lesser degree, in South-East and western Asia. Conflict zones, even if they are receiving food aid, tend to be food poor. Social and climatic disaster usually combine to create situations of resource poverty that set the stage for chronic food poverty for years to come.

Seasonal or periodic hunger constitutes the second general case of food shortage. This persists outside conflict zones in local settings where food production combined with other economic activities is insufficient to support adequate diets year-round or from year to year where single-year productivity is variable and low. Increasingly, these pockets of food shortfall are reached by intervention programmes that provide relief food, often through "food-for-work" employment programmes. Where markets or food relief penetrate relatively isolated local food systems, as in many parts of Africa and South Asia, food shortage is removed but is replaced by chronic food poverty (Messer 1989).

Food poverty

The main factors influencing food poverty are shortage (especially related to conflict), entitlement strategies that are not sufficiently remunerative and diversified, and macroeconomic policies, especially the early stages of structural adjustment, that make food and other services less affordable.

Proportionately more food-poor households exist in food-short regions, but adequate food in a region does not guarantee freedom from hunger. Undiversified production; low food prices for rural produce relative to other commodities; excessive taxation; lack of transport and market facilities; and lack of control over land, labour, wages, and prices – all contribute to households being unable to meet their own needs. Food poverty is most severe in sub-Saharan Africa, largely because of shortage. It poses enormous problems also in most countries of Asia and Latin America, where aggregate food supply should be sufficient but severe inequalities persist in income and food distribution.

Within urban areas, underemployment and underremuneration contribute to incapacities to meet food needs although, in urban areas, subsidized food, health care, and other compensatory services tend to be more available. Food poverty is greater in rural areas, which tend to be more at risk of being excluded from government social services and safety nets should crops and income strategies fail.

Income diversification is usually cited as one of the "solutions" for food poverty. Those with multiple income streams tend to be less at risk of hunger when any of the streams fails. But transitions often constitute potential hazards as well. Since the 1980s, analysts observe that those households experiencing transition economies, which are in the process of shifting from subsistence to cash-cropping and other sources of income, and from customary kinship and community to state-organized safety nets, may be more vulnerable to hunger. In addition, those countries undergoing economic (structural) adjustment may be more vulnerable: they need special anti-poverty and social programmes to avoid intolerable and conflict-potentiating food poverty.

In both urban and rural areas, food-poor households experience synergisms between malnutrition, illness, and unhealthy environment that reduce well-being and increase hunger. Meta-analysis of the sources of child mortality indicate that even mild-to-moderate malnutrition potentiates child mortality from infectious disease (Pelletier 1994). Household poverty restricts access to both nutrition and health care.

Food deprivation

Chapter 5 examined issues of intra-household distribution of food – whether the burden of food poverty is shared equally among household members, and also what types of individuals are likely to suffer from food deprivation in the absence of food poverty. Significant variables are gender and age. Pregnant and lactating women are generally the most vulnerable to hunger because they have elevated nutritional needs that may or may not be perceived and that, for cultural as well as economic reasons, are likely to go unmet in food-poor (but also not so poor) households. Analysts point out that estimates of female nutritional needs (requirements) often incorporate gender bias: they assume smaller body size and therefore lower nutritional needs, and also tend to underestimate women's physical activities and caloric expenditures. These underestimates operate to reduce expected and standard nutrient intakes of females from very young ages. Additionally, the extra nutritional requirement for pregnant and lactating women deserves greater emphasis: women in the developing world still spend much of their adult lives in these reproductive states with their heightened nutritional needs.

Geographically, the problem of reproductive-aged women's malnutrition is most pronounced in parts of India and neighbouring countries in South Asia. Children in South Asia and South-East Asia, and in pockets in sub-Saharan Africa, also experience elevated risk of vitamin A- and iodine-deficiency diseases. Reproductive-aged women the world over are at risk for iron deficiency. Even as women appear to be getting greater access to food calories, as shown in the Indian data provided in this volume, they still may not be getting their fair share of micronutrients and other high-quality foods, and this affects their well-being, fertility, and longevity.

Nutrition incorporates notions of food, health, and care, any of which may or may not show gender bias. Food-energy-intake data are mixed, especially for Africa and Asia, where apparent patterns of both male and female bias coexist in different national samples. The conventional wisdom, that females are less well nourished than males because they encounter discrimination in food allocation, does not always conform to the evidence: counter-evidence is accumulating from Africa, where females tend to be more autonomous and economically active; contrary evidence is also emerging from South and South-East Asia. Anti-female discrimination in food-energy intakes, where staple foods are relatively affordable, appears less than expected. Food poverty, moreover, does not appear to be the main determinant of preferential feeding of males over females: positive male-gender bias in India appears to operate more forcefully in households that have more, not fewer, resources.

Gender differences in age-specific survival persist in the face of this seemingly contradictory evidence. Accumulating evidence indicates that bias is less likely to occur as a result of differences in food (energy) distribution than it is as a result of differences in health-care allocation. Skewed male survivorship, plus ethnographic evidence, suggest that males, indeed, are favoured in expenditures for health care. They may also be favoured in consumption of luxury foods, rich in protein and micronutrients. This interpretation is supported also in recent anthropological studies of South Asia and South America that found evidence of anti-female gender bias in health care and survival but mixed data on gender-skewing in food intake (Messer 1997). Whereas food energy may be relatively inexpensive and accessible as a result of agricultural improvement programmes and government safety nets, health care may be more available but less accessible to poor households, which therefore may ration use to (male) members who are considered to be more valuable economically or socially over their lifetimes.

Evidence of nutritional discrimination against infants and young children also contains errors due to data-collection bias or omissions. The authors point out that many countries omit breastmilk from records of food intake of very young children, so of course they appear to be horrendously undernourished! Reports of infant intakes that leave out breastmilk, and children's diets that refer to absolute intakes instead of intakes relative to gender-based standards, appear to account for some proportion of such biases communicated in the literature. However, these revised interpretations of the data on energy intakes must be accepted with caution and extremely important qualifications. Breast-fed children may still be moderately or severely underfed relative to their needs. Female children may still suffer life-threatening discrimination in allocations of health and other types of care, as well as of higher-quality nutrient-rich foods. These new data and interpretations suggest that food-energy biases are less common even in Indian regions of endemic excess female mortality, but they do not contradict the indirect evidence – appalling excess female mortality – of anti-female bias. Indian women need to have access to better health care and higher-nutrient-density foods, particularly during their reproductive years. Households and individuals, in cases of the better-off households, need education about nutritional needs and the value of women's health and work; poorer households also need additional economic resources.

Policy implications

Food and nutrition policies tend to be either short (5–10 years) or medium (20–50 years) term and to have measurable versus general programmatic goals. We connect here two recent plans to reduce world hunger to our hunger typology and analysis.

The Bellagio Declaration: "Overcoming Hunger in the 1990s"

A significant short-term effort to identify what could be done for hunger by the end of the decade was "Overcoming Hunger in the 1990s." This international NGO effort, promulgated as a Bellagio Declaration in 1989, aimed to reduce half the world's hunger in 10 years. It introduced a focused but multi-faceted scheme that set four achievable (measurable) goals: (1) to end famine deaths, especially by moving food into zones of armed conflict; (2) to end hunger in half the world's poorest households; (3) to eliminate at least half the hunger of women and children by expanding maternal child health coverage; and (4) to eliminate vitamin A and iodine deficiencies as public health problems. The Bellagio Declaration also affirmed food as a human right, and insisted that progress will come only through the joint efforts and energies of grass-roots and community organizations combined with state and international agencies. A five-year report concluded that progress was being made on all except the first goal: conflict continued to be an intractable problem. Progress reported for China, Indonesia, and Thailand contributed to the global downward trend in numbers malnourished and to meeting the "halfway" goals to halve hunger. The mid-decade assessment also suggested that additional investments in women's education and health, clean water, infrastructure, and community organizing would go far toward eliminating hunger in the future (Messer and Uvin 1996). In short, the report, while hopeful, was far from complacent.

"2020 Vision for Food, Agriculture, and the Environment"

The "2020 Vision for Food, Agriculture, and the Environment" initiated by the International Food Policy Research Institute (IFPRI) in 1994, aimed to set medium-term priorities and actions to avert a future world food crisis. Concept background papers assembled opposing views on pertinent issues such as ecological resources, population, trade, poverty, and nutrition. The goal of the series was to develop a consensus, among the many parties concerned about world food and nutrition, on a global plan of action to secure adequate food, healthy populations, and sustainable environment for the next century.

Overall, the 2020 project offered a diverse menu of actions that might be taken to prevent food shortage, prevent food insecurity, and meet the nutritional health needs of all the world's people. In their series of six "priority areas for action," number one was "Strengthen the capacity of developing country governments to perform appropriate functions" (IFPRI 1995: 23), which involves both more effective action by governments (in partnership with other sectors) in policy-making and implementation, and also the prerequisite of "improved security and personal safety." Specific actions include giving priority to conflict resolution and prevention in areas where armed conflicts and civil strife are occurring or are imminent. National and international development agencies need to incorporate conflict prevention into programme and project planning, by identifying and then targeting for intervention those areas where the potential for conflict is high, and defusing them by delivering aid in manners that avoid competition and that foster (or demand) cooperation among groups or communities. Conventionally, agricultural research focused on areas of high growth potential, especially when implementing Green Revolution seed–water–fertilizer technologies

186

that were dependent on good soils and reliable water supply. The 2020 report recommends that the very poorest or seemingly hopeless areas also receive special priority, as these may be areas of high conflict potential; resources should be directed toward these areas that are conflict prone, by finding and promoting "engines of growth" that might overcome and move people beyond perceived scarcities and thereby preclude disruptive and destructive negative growth that has characterized conflict areas over the past three decades.

Other recommendations addressed issues such as more secure agricultural production in manners that promote rural livelihoods and protect environment, aspects of ecological management, and ways to create more efficient and effective markets for agricultural inputs and outputs. A separate recommendation was to improve productivity and health of low-income people, who also need increased access to employment and productive assets.

This vision focuses on sustainable food supply to meet nutritional and environmental goals for the next century. It attempts to expand the agricultural agenda at the same time that it tries not to depart too greatly from its principal mission theme of "food." It leaves priorities to regions or countries.

Synthesis

Key points of contact between these policy exercises and the hunger typology are their recognition of the need for greater cooperation between the different sectors of society that potentially impact on food policy, their focus on conflict and conflict prevention, and their emphasis on improving the lives and livelihoods of women. The policy exercises also share a common concern that, although the world is in crisis, there are already many tools to help prevent and relieve further suffering. Both exercises urge support for legal mechanisms to promote people's right to adequate food and nutrition.

Analysis of hunger situations provides guidance for policy makers to map nutritional suffering in time and space for more effective action. Recent world summits on environment, population, social development, and food all emphasize the potential for better mapping of vulnerable regions, communities, and households. This is, in part, a technical recommendation. They also emphasize the need for a stabler political environment in which diagnosis of, and response to, hunger problems can take place. Hunger situations ultimately are amenable to political solutions, much as their existence and persistence are due to political causes. International committees, which seem to be gaining both political wisdom and technological expertise, still need to acquire greater political will to act.

Works cited

International Food Policy Research Institute (IFPRI). 1995. *A 2020 Vision for Food, Agriculture, and the Environment. The Vision, Challenge, and Recommended Action*. Washington, D.C.: IFPRI.

Messer, Ellen. 1989. "Seasonality in Food Systems: An Anthropological Perspective on Household Food Security." In: D. Sahn, ed. *Seasonal Variability in Third World Agriculture: The Consequences for Food Security*. Baltimore: Johns Hopkins University Press, pp. 151–175.

———. 1997. "Intrahousehold Allocation of Food and Health Care. Recent Anthropological Findings and Understandings." *Social Science and Medicine* 44, No. 11: 1675–1684.

———, and Peter Uvin, eds. 1995. *The Hunger Report: 1995*. Amsterdam: Gordon & Breach.

Pelletier, David. (1994). "The Potentiating Effects of Malnutrition on Child Mortality: Epidemiological Evidence and Policy Implications." *Nutrition Reviews* 52, No. 12: 409–415.

Uvin, Peter. 1996. "The State of World Hunger." In: E. Messer and P. Uvin, eds. *The Hunger Report: 1995*. Amsterdam: Gordon & Breach, pp. 1–18.

Index

191